TIRED
OF BEING
TIRED

Other books by Dr. Michael A. Schmidt:

Beyond Antibiotics

Managing the Patient with Chronic Fatigue

Childhood Ear Infections

TIRED
OF BEING
TIRED

*Achieving
Peak Energy
& Mental Clarity*

Dr. Michael A. Schmidt

Frog, Ltd.
Berkeley, California

Tired of Being Tired: Overcoming Chronic Fatigue and Low Energy

Copyright © 1995 by Michael A. Schmidt. No portion of this book, except for brief review, may be reproduced in any form without written permission of the publisher. For information contact Frog, Ltd. c/o North Atlantic Books.

Published by Frog, Ltd.

Frog, Ltd. books are distributed by
North Atlantic Books
P.O. Box 12327
Berkeley, California 94712

Cover and book design by Paula Morrison
Typeset by Catherine Campaigne

Printed in the United States of America by Malloy Lithographing

Library of Congress Cataloging-in-Publication Data
Schmidt, Michael A., 1958–
    Tired of being tired : overcoming chronic fatigue and low energy / Michael
Schmidt.
        p.   cm.
    Includes bibliographical references and index.
    ISBN 1-883319-16-1
        1. Fatigue.   2. Chronic fatigue syndrome.   3. Fatigue—Etiology.   I. Title
        [DNLM: 1. Fatigue—diagnosis.   2. Fatigue Syndrome, Chronic—
diagnosis.   3. Fatigue—therapy.   4. Fatigue Syndrome, Chronic—
therapy.   WB 146 S353t   1994]
    RB150.F37S35   1994
    616'.047—dc20
    DNLM/DLC
    for Library of Congress   93-48676
                                                                                        CIP

3   4   5   6   7   8   9 / 03   02   01   00   99

To my teachers in the ways of the heart,
Caleb and Julian

A Note to Readers

THIS BOOK HAS been written as a guide to those who suffer from fatigue, low vitality, and chronic tiredness. The reader should understand that there are many factors that may contribute to fatigue. Fatigue can be due to simple factors such as insufficient physical activity or to more serious illness such as cancer or heart disease. This book is an attempt to describe many common causes of fatigue and to suggest possible remedies. Since fatigue can be a result of serious medical problems, it is important that you report your symptoms to your doctor and follow up with the appropriate tests and treatment. This guide can serve as a helpful tool for you and your doctor to uncover the cause of your fatigue. Before undertaking any of the recommendations provided in this book, it is advisable to consult your personal doctor.

This book is based on my clinical experience and on the most recent scientific research. However, as with any endeavor, do not merely accept my interpretation of the evidence as fact. Review the relevant research, explore other resources, and come to your own conclusions. This book should serve as a resource and a guide, not the final authority. Also recognize that researchers are working feverishly to understand the factors that contribute to chronic fatigue. In this regard, new evidence may either confirm or replace many of the concepts presented here.

Acknowledgements

I WOULD LIKE to thank my friends, colleagues, students, and others who have helped influence my course in the healing arts. To those who shared their thoughtful insights that have helped in the preparation of this book, I am especially grateful: William Crook, M.D., Jon Pangborn, Ph.D., Andy Bralley, Ph.D., Jeffrey Bland, Ph.D., Paul Westby, D.C., Thomas Miller, D.C., Joseph Sweere, D.C., Gary Osborn, R.Ph., David Perlmutter, M.D., Keith Sehnert, M.D., Russell Jaffe, M.D., Luke Bucci, Ph.D., Sidney Baker, M.D., Larry Dossey, M.D., Steven Gresham, and Shannon Dufresne.

I am grateful to Kathy Glass and Paula Morrison who put their artistic and editorial touches on this book. Their efforts helped give clarity and consistency.

I would especially like to thank my wife, Julie. She is always supportive, thoughtful, and patient as I scurry through the world of research, teaching, writing, and deadlines.

Table of Contents

Part II: Steps to Improved Energy

Foreword

As this century comes to a close, health care providers are being overwhelmed by an ever growing number of patients who, because of chronic lack of energy, find themselves unable to fully engage in a meaningful life experience. It is perhaps this group of patients, more than any other, that poses the greatest challenge to the modern Western medical paradigm. The Newtonian billiard ball germ-theory model typically relied upon by Western medical science to explain our maladies quite clearly fails us when we are engaged by these patients to unravel their protean complaints.

Patients who are chronically fatigued do not suffer from a specific disease entity. Medical students do not learn about chronic fatigue between the cancer and cystitis chapters of their medical books. That is because chronic fatigue is not an "it" like tuberculosis or bunions. What is so unique and perplexing about chronically fatigued patients are the incredibly varied roads they have taken to arrive at their Rome of disability. Herein lies one of the fundamental mysteries to understanding the chronically fatigued patient which is so well explored in these pages. Dr. Schmidt, in this book, first delineates and defines the various pathways leading to the condition of generalized fatigue, typically in association with immune dysfunction. It is only through careful attention to these factors that health care provider and patient alike will be able to create a treatment protocol designed to recreate internal harmony and rekindle an energetic feeling of well being.

Chronically fatigued patients clearly represent a challenge to the health care provider. Their problems do not lend themselves to the quick fix, their pains are not easily pacified, their histories and previous medical records may take hours to digest, and their questions may, at times, seem unending. Nevertheless, with careful attention paid to understanding *who is the patient who has the disease* as opposed to *what is the disease that this patient has,* health care practitioners will gain satisfaction by developing successful treatment programs exploiting each patient's uniqueness.

After considering the various causative factors and curative options offered in this book, one is left to consider disease prevention. As stated by the Yellow Emperor in the second century B.C., "Prevention is the ultimate principle of wisdom. To cure a disease after it has manifest is like digging a well when one already feels thirsty, or forging weapons when the war has already begun." This is where this book may have its most meaningful impact. As we consider the profound influence that attention to nutrition, vitamins, careful use of antibiotics, exercise, and so many other factors presented in these pages have on maintaining good health, we realize that prevention is an ultimate principle of wisdom.

David Perlmutter, M.D.
Neurology and Preventive Medicine
Naples Neurological Associates
Naples, Florida

Introduction

FOR SEVERAL YEARS I have toured the country lecturing to health professionals about managing patients with chronic fatigue. As I began to get feedback from doctors, it occurred to me that there was little information available to the general public about helpful ways to understand and remedy chronic fatigue. There are many good books on the subject of chronic fatigue syndrome. But this disorder truly only effects a small percentage of people who are fatigued. My approach has been to look at the bigger picture of chronic fatigue and identify its many faces. This is what we have been teaching medical professionals and it was the subject of the study guide Managing the Patient with Chronic Fatigue. *Tired of Being Tired* began as this teaching guide for health professionals. It has evolved into what I believe is a valuable guide for anyone concerned with fatigue and low vitality.

Humans are extremely complex beings. Any attempt to suggest we have all the answers to the mystery of fatigue is beyond reason. In this book I have identified many factors that give rise to fatigue. You may find many helpful solutions in this book which will help you overcome your fatigue. However, there will always be people who have more complex illnesses resistant to these treatments. For those, this book may provide insight and alert you to avenues of assessment and treatment that your doctors may not have investigated.

How to Use This Book

This book is written with two purposes in mind. First, the information presented may help you identify the nature of your fatigue.

Some of the suggested strategies may be sufficiently helpful that you overcome your fatigue—and win the battle. For others it may not be so simple. My second purpose is to give those who have unsuccessfully sought help for their fatigue hope, a different viewpoint, and information that they can assimilate that will perhaps start them on a new course. Much of this business of being a patient means doing your homework and giving your doctor all the information about your condition that you can. In some cases you may need the courage to explore other kinds of doctors or treatments foreign to a specific physician you have chosen.

Each chapter describes specific factors that contribute to fatigue. These subdivisions provide more detailed information that can help you clarify the cause of your own fatigue. The subheadings include the following:

Introduction. The introduction contains background information about the subject being discussed whether it be nutritional deficiency, sleep disorders, or something else. It is meant to give basic information about a topic. The Introduction is an overview.

Signs and Symptoms. Each chapter shows the most common signs and symptoms associated with an illness, deficiency, or exposure. Use this as a guide to learn whether you might suffer from this problem. However, note that many conditions have symptoms that overlap. Symptoms alone are a helpful guide, but are not definitive.

Laboratory Tests. Each section contains a discussion of tests your doctor may order. What is unique about this section is that it contains some tests with which your doctor may be unfamiliar. For instance, there are tests to measure whether toxic exposure might be the cause of your fatigue. There are also tests for vitamins and mineral status. There are urine tests that look at the energy-producing pathways of your metabolism. There are tests for amino acids that can affect brain neurotransmitters and myriad other aspects of body chemistry. In these and other instances, the tests can be highly revealing.

I also show which tests commonly used in medical offices are not accurate in identifying the problem they seek to identify. For example, the *serum* test for magnesium is not ideal for detecting magnesium deficiency. There are better tests, which I will describe. The serum test for vitamin B_{12} is likewise not as good at discovering deficiency as other tests.

Treatment. Each treatment section describes some of the common medical treatments, but focuses on healing methods from the perspective of integrated or holistic medicine. These, again, are to be considered overviews since each subject is more complex than the depth of this book allows.

In Review. Each chapter closes with a brief review of the key points in that chapter. This will help you recall the highlights and serve as a quick reference should you want to go back and review later.

A Note about Cause and Effect

In this and many other books, authors talk about causes of this or that phenomenon. I have attempted to minimize use of the word "cause" because it is very difficult to determine cause and effect. Some medical systems such as traditional Chinese Medicine and homeopathic medicine have complex, systemic concepts of cause and effect. These systems describe patterns of disharmony or disrupted function, which cannot be related to a single cause.

Certainly there are factors that can be causative. An automobile accident that results in a neck injury is causative. A chemical burn is causative. Poor energy may be "caused" by vitamin B_{12} deficiency. Yet, when we are talking about fatigue, there are so many factors at work that the word "cause" often seems inappropriate. Thus, when you find the word cause in this book, it is meant loosely.

The reader should know that this book addresses a variety of health concerns in an overview fashion. Each of the topics discussed are the subject of intensive medical investigation and have lengthy books written about them. In this regard, this book should not be considered the final word on any of the subjects covered. If you suspect your problem may lie specifically in one of the categories discussed, see your doctor and consult the appropriate resources for more information.

Dr. Michael A. Schmidt

Part I

Tired of Being Tired

Chapter 1

The Many Faces of Fatigue

SOMETHING ISN'T QUITE RIGHT. Modern technology was supposed to make our lives so much easier that we would merely work a little and spend the abundant free time pursuing our favorite leisure activity. Unfortunately, we seem to be working harder, working longer hours, playing less, and certainly not lying on the beach watching the clouds roll by. Our fast-paced, rapid-fire modern life seems to leave many of us breathless—as though we can never accomplish all we would like, as though there is never enough time, and for some, as though *there is not enough energy* to get it all done.

For millions of people in Western society, chronic fatigue, tiredness, and low vitality seem to be the bane of twentieth-century existence. Indeed, fatigue, tiredness, and low vitality are the most common symptoms for which people seek medical care. A recent survey found that 24 percent of adults patronizing primary care clinics "always feel tired."[1]

Why is it that so many people complain of fatigue and low energy? Why is chronic fatigue so common? What causes chronic tiredness and low energy? Am I tired because of something I eat? Am I deficient in vitamins? Is there something in the environment causing my fatigue? Do I have a serious disease? Why can't my doctor find the cause of my poor energy level? What is this new disease called chronic fatigue syndrome? Do I have it? How do I know? How could I find out? What can I do about it if I do have it?

This is just a sample of questions commonly asked by people who are fatigued. The degree of fatigue ranges from those who just don't have the energy they would like to those who are so debilitated they cannot work or function, spending much of their time resting in bed. This book is for both of you.

Fatigue has many faces and many causes. Fatigue and tiredness mean different things to different people. To a mother with three young children, fatigue may mean exhaustion and a feeling of never being able to get enough done. To a workaholic businessman, fatigue may mean getting up sluggish every morning and being unproductive for half the day. To an athlete, fatigue may mean poor recovery or lack of competitive drive. For someone else, it may mean confusion or inability to concentrate. Whatever your definition of fatigue and your personal experience, there are answers. The key is asking the right questions and knowing where to look.

A disorder called chronic fatigue syndrome (CFS), post-viral fatigue syndrome (PVFS), or chronic fatigue immune dysfunction syndrome (CFIDS) has received an enormous amount of media attention lately and is the subject of several excellent books. Unfortunately, this has caused many people who suffer from fatigue and low energy to believe they suffer from chronic fatigue *syndrome* when they do not. Moreover, it has caused many doctors to roll their eyes at patients who come in with another "disease of the month."

Before we go any further you should understand an important distinction that will be an underlying assumption of this entire book: Not all people who suffer from chronic fatigue and low energy suffer from chronic fatigue *syndrome*. Chronic fatigue *syndrome* is a real disorder that causes an enormous amount of suffering and disability. Researchers around the world are working diligently to unravel the mystery of chronic fatigue *syndrome*. But most researchers will admit that chronic fatigue *syndrome* only affects about five to ten percent of those people who complain of chronic fatigue, tiredness, and low vitality.

I have italicized *syndrome* repeatedly in this chapter so you understand that chronic fatigue *syndrome* and generalized chronic fatigue
are usually separate entities. However, chronic fatigue *syndrome* is
often an outgrowth of some of the same factors that cause general
fatigue and low vitality.

According to a 1994 Vancouver, B.C. consensus conference on
chronic fatigue syndrome, the following criteria should be met to
qualify for a diagnosis of chronic fatigue syndrome. (Note that the
definition is continually being revised as we learn more.)

A. Fatigue

   Severe, unexplained fatigue that is not relieved by rest,
   which can cause disability and which has an identifiable
   onset (i.e., not lifelong fatigue).

B. Four or more of the following symptoms.

   1. Memory and concentration problems

   2. Sore throat

   3. Tender lymph nodes

   4. Arthralgia (joint pain)

   5. Myalgia (muscle pain)

   6. Headaches

   7. Non-refreshing sleep

   8. Post-exertional malaise

C. Exclusions

   People may be excluded if they have an active medical
   diagnosis, a previous non-resolved medical diagnosis,
   physical findings suggesting either of the first two,
   melancholic/psychologic depression, eating disorders,
   psychosis, alcohol/substance abuse, or severe obesity.[2]

As you can probably see, most people who are chronically tired
do not fit these criteria. But even if the criteria are met, one must
still go about the business of determining the cause. This book is an
attempt to help you by explaining the many factors that might be

contributing to your fatigue and giving suggestions about how you might go about solving the riddle. According to Paul Cheney, M.D., a leading chronic fatigue syndrome physician and researcher, some people with *severe* chronic fatigue syndrome paradoxically become worse when following the same treatment regimen that makes other patients with less severe chronic fatigue syndrome better. For this reason, it is vital that a patient with CFS embark on a treatment plan with great care and under the guidance of a doctor knowledgeable in treating severe chronic fatigue syndrome. Here is a preview of some of the factors that cause or are associated with fatigue and low vitality.

Vitamin insufficiency	Mineral insufficiency
Food allergy/intolerance	Chemical toxicity
Blood sugar problems	Thyroid trouble
Overweight/underlean	Elevated blood fats
Irritable bowel syndrome	Poor sleep/insomnia
Physical inactivity	Overtraining in athletes
Antibiotic overuse	Fibromyalgia
Depression	Stress
Overuse of prescription drugs	Hidden infections
Cancer	Heart disease
Lung disease	Inadequate light

My goal is to help you with the detective work of finding the culprits in your fatigue and to point you squarely in the direction of improved energy and vitality.

How Energy Is Produced in Your Body and Why You May Not Have Enough

Throughout this book I will talk about energy. People who are fatigued or tired complain of a lack of energy. "Doctor, why am I so tired?" and "Doctor, I just don't have the energy to do what I want," are typical laments. The patient and the doctor define energy in slightly different ways. To the patient, having energy means having the zip available to get up and do things. It means being able to sustain a certain amount of effort without getting tired. To the doctor, energy also refers to the biochemical processes that go on inside cells that are devoted to the production of a substance called ATP. ATP stands for adenosine triphosphate. But if you wish, you can think of ATP as **A T**hing of **P**ower, since that's essentially what ATP is. I'll just tell you briefly about ATP so you can understand why nutritional therapy is so important in treating people who are fatigued. It will also help you understand why toxins in the environment can contribute to fatigue.

ATP is a high-energy substance produced in millions of little power-packed structures called mitochondria. Each second your body produces billions of molecules of ATP. They live for only a fraction of a second and are then regenerated. If your ATP production is low, your body doesn't produce enough energy to function at its peak. Some people with chronic fatigue produce ATP so inefficiently that they have only enough energy to keep their basic body processes going.

Your body can make ATP from protein, fat, and carbohydrate. In order to do so it requires vitamins and minerals such as niacin, riboflavin, pantothenic acid, magnesium, and so on. When these are not present in sufficient amounts, your energy-producing machinery does not work properly and ATP is not produced as efficiently. The effect—low energy and fatigue. All of the body's detoxication systems also require ATP. If your body harbors chemical toxins, not only can the chemicals themselves bind ATP, but once the ATP is depleted it is unable to stimulate other detoxication reactions. In short, chemical toxins block energy production directly and make it more difficult for you to eliminate toxins in the future—a vicious cycle.

An analogy may help explain the interaction between nutrients and energy (ATP). In our analogy you might liken the body to an automobile. To make a car go you need gasoline (the fuel), spark plugs (the spark), and an ignition or starter. When you turn the key in the ignition an electric current is sent through the spark plugs. An arc of electricity leaps across the gap in the part of the spark plug located in the cylinder where a tiny amount of gasoline is injected.

When the gasoline and the spark interact, a small explosion takes place in the cylinder that makes the piston move. This drives the crank shaft which ultimately makes the car move.

You can have a tankful of gas and a large engine, but if your spark plugs are gummed up there is no way to ignite the gasoline. With no way to ignite the gasoline the engine does not run. Now, rarely are all spark plugs bad at once, so let's assume that only two of six are bad. In this case, some of the spark plugs ignite to burn some of the gasoline, but the engine sputters, spits, and does not run at its peak. It does not make full use of the potential power that exists. It does not generate the same amount of energy from a given amount of fuel. We call this not running on all cylinders, a car's version of fatigue. The body is the same way. You may have more than enough fuel in the form of protein, fat, and carbohydrate. (In fact, most people do.) But if the vitamins and minerals are not present in adequate amounts, the pathways of energy metabolism sputter and spit and only churn out a limited number of ATP units. The body does not make use of the full energy potential that exists by virtue of the amount of fuel you have. Our comparison might look like this:

Fuel/gasoline = protein, fat, carbohydrate from diet
Ignition = vitamin and mineral co-factors that trigger the enzymes to activate
Spark plugs = enzymes that convert one compound to another

Without the ignition the spark plugs just sit dormant. Likewise, without the co-factor vitamins and minerals the enzymes are not activated. You can see there are many limiting factors.

Another factor to consider in energy production is the size of the engine. Our engine for energy metabolism just happens to be muscle. In fact, the little power-packed mitochondria that make ATP (energy) are more concentrated in muscle than in any other tissue. The more muscle you have the better you will be at converting your dietary fuel into energy.

If you have more body fat relative to muscle, you essentially have a smaller engine (muscle) with more fuel (fat) to burn. If you add a five-gallon gas tank to a lawn mower engine, is the engine more powerful? If you add a 20-gallon tank to a lawn mower engine, does it make it more powerful? The answer, of course, is "no." This is one reason weight loss programs that do not incorporate exercise ultimately never go anywhere. They never increase the size of the "engine" necessary to burn the fuel.

To carry our analogy a bit further, what happens when the gasoline tank gets water inside? It makes it impossible for the spark plugs to ignite the gasoline. Chemicals in the environment have a similar effect on the production of ATP. They prevent energy from being efficiently produced in the cell from the fuel. Chemicals can bind with co-factor nutrients, rendering them useless, and they can actually bind with ATP itself, making it unavailable. We'll see later how such events happen with magnesium and aluminum.

One reason I believe many doctors are frustrated treating patients with chronic fatigue is they do not consider nutritional biochemistry or environmental factors. They may not understand the effect nutrient deficiency has on energy metabolism. They may not understand how heavy metals and pesticides can block energy production in the cell and therefore in the entire body. Giving a patient with disordered energy metabolism due to nutrient deficiency a prescription drug to control symptoms can be likened to putting "stop leak" in your radiator to prevent the leakage of radiator fluid. You will eventually need to repair the radiator.

There is one final distinction to note before we continue. That is, health and disease exist on a continuum. We are not healthy one minute and sick the next (unless, perhaps, we've been in an accident). The progression from optimal health to disease is a gradual descent that passes through phases. The descent can take many years and involve many stressors. Likewise, the road back to optimum health is a continuum that takes time.

Health ←—→ Dysfunction ←—→ Disease ←—→ Disintegration

In the following chapters, we will focus on the factors that contribute to fatigue, tiredness, and low vitality and help you chart a course for solving your fatigue dilemma. To begin this journey, we will look into the digestive process, since the gastrointestinal tract is so central to the development of fatigue.

In Review

1. Chronic fatigue, tiredness, and low vitality affect millions of people.
2. Chronic fatigue and chronic fatigue *syndrome* are not the same.
3. Chronic fatigue can have many faces and may be due to many different factors.
4. Energy production in the body is focused on production of energy-containing compounds such as ATP.
5. ATP can be prevented from forming by nutritional insufficiency, chemical toxins, poor muscle mass, and other factors.
6. To optimize energy production we want to optimize vitamin and mineral intake, and take in adequate protein (5 to 20 percent of total calories), fat (15 to 20 percent of total calories), and carbohydrate (65 percent of total calories).
7. To optimize the use of our dietary fuel for energy production we want to have a high lean body mass, meaning more muscle and less fat. Remember, *muscle is the engine.*
8. Health and disease exist on a continuum.

Chapter 2

Intestinal Problems

MANY DIFFERENT FACTORS that contribute to chronic fatigue can be traced back to problems in the intestinal tract. To more clearly show why, it is important to give a brief background on the critical steps of digestion and assimilation.

The digestive process begins in your head, with your choice of food and your state of mind while eating. Once you've made your choice and put the food in your mouth, the salivary glands secrete enzymes that begin to digest carbohydrates (sugars, starches). Proper chewing is also needed to ensure that the food is sufficiently ground when it reaches the stomach. The stomach secretes hydrochloric acid and pepsin, which begin to digest proteins and serve to acidify the mass (bolus) of food for delivery to the small intestine. The stomach also exerts a powerful grinding action on the food.

Once the acidic mixture of food reaches the duodenum (upper part of the small intestine), it triggers the release of the hormones cholecystokinin and secretin, which (respectively) stimulate contraction of the gall bladder and the secretion of pancreatic juices. The gall bladder releases compounds that help in the emulsification and absorption of fats. The pancreatic juices contain bicarbonate (like baking soda) and enzymes. The bicarbonate raises the pH of the duodenum enough to activate the pancreatic digestive enzymes.

These enzymes break down protein, fat, and carbohydrate into smaller, more absorbable units.

As the mass of food moves down the middle section of the intestinal tract (jejunum) it no longer contains the crude, bound elements of food such as protein, carbohydrate, and fat. It now contains a mixture of amino acids, small protein fragments, chylomicrons (fats), vitamins, minerals, and other substances. The nutrients essential to optimum health are then absorbed into the small intestine and transported to the liver, where they are packaged, processed, stored, and utilized for the billions of activities that drive the human body.

Meanwhile, undigestible and unabsorbable material continues its transit into the large intestine (colon) through a gate known as the ileocecal valve. The material that enters here includes bile salts, cholesterol, undigested meat and vegetable fibers, dead intestinal cells (which are replaced every three days), and other materials. Once past the ileocecal valve, the mass of "waste" reaches the colon, home to billions of microorganisms (bacteria, yeast, etc.). The colon is primarily responsible for reabsorbing water back into the body. However, the organisms that live here are highly active and do their best to further digest (for themselves) the food residues that pass their way, and manufacture vitamins and beneficial fatty acids.

Finally, the material moves through the colon to be eliminated as feces. Feces is really a collection of billions of microorganisms (bacteria, yeast, etc.), short-chain fatty acids, long-chain fatty acids, cholesterol, enzymes, and undigested food residue (fiber, etc.).

Any point in the digestive process can be disrupted, which can affect how you digest and assimilate nutrients. As you will see, nutrient sufficiency is a critical consideration in chronic fatigue. Below is a list of some of the factors that can disrupt the digestive process. (Note that at every stage there are numerous factors and medical conditions that may have an adverse influence.)

1. *Mood, mind.* Eating while reading, agitated, hurried, or stressed causes lower levels of digestive enzymes to be produced.

2. *Improper chewing,* which is very common, inadequately grinds the food so the nutrients are not as thoroughly extracted.

3. *Insufficient hydrochloric acid (HCl)* leads to insufficient early-stage protein breakdown in the stomach and insufficient acid to stimulate the pancreatic enzymes. Insufficient HCl is common in modern cultures, especially with the high consumption of antacids. If the pH (or acidity) is not correct in the stomach, it affects the pH throughout the entire digestive tract.

4. *Pancreatic enzyme insufficiency* prevents adequate breakdown of protein, fat, and carbohydrate into their constituent amino acids, vitamins, minerals, essential fatty acids, and simple sugars. When pancreatic enzymes are not adequate, nutrient insufficiency is very common.

5. *Inflammation of the small intestine lining.* This can occur as a result of years of poor dietary choices, antibiotic overuse, antiinflammatory drug use, intestinal infection, psychological stress, excessive alcohol consumption, food allergy, malnutrition, radiation therapy, chemotherapy, nutrient insufficiency, environmental toxins, intestinal toxins, and malabsorption. When the lining of the intestine is inflamed, nutrient transport into the bloodstream does not occur properly.

6. *Overgrowth of intestinal bacteria (dysbiosis),* leading to a toxic bowel. This is described later. When dysbiosis occurs, food residue that reaches the colon can be acted upon by the "unfriendly" organisms that live there. These organisms can turn the food material into toxins such as aldehydes and alcohol that influence the brain and energy production. Some are even converted into cancer-causing substances. Some unfriendly gut organisms even break the bonds of conjugated estrogen and cause estrogens that were tagged for elimination to be re-released back into the bloodstream. This can alter hormonal cycles. In fact, some women who suffer from PMS improve by correcting their intestinal ecology.

7. *Altered transit time.* The food you eat should move from your mouth through the intestines and be eliminated as feces within a twelve- to eighteen-hour period. If the time is shorter or longer, it suggests intestinal problems. Longer transit times give the intestinal bacteria more time to ferment or putrefy the intestinal contents into not-so-friendly byproducts. The putrefactive or fermentative byprod-

ucts can be reabsorbed into the bloodstream and interfere with metabolism, energy production, immunity, and other functions.

In chapter 14, I note that chronic antibiotic use is a common precipitating factor in many people with chronic fatigue. Antibiotics
trigger poor health because their excessive use can seriously disrupt
digestion, absorption, assimilation. The dysbiosis they create leads
to the production of toxins in the bowel that can be reabsorbed into
the body and act as immunotoxins, neurotoxins, and hepatotoxins,
affecting many body systems.

Laboratory Tests

There are many tests that can be used to assess intestinal function.
I will discuss just a few here, one of which can be done at home.

• *CDSA.* The comprehensive digestive stool analysis (Great Smokies Diagnostic Laboratory, Asheville, North Carolina; Meridian Valley Laboratory, Kent, Washington) is a stool test that evaluates 24
different parameters of intestinal function such as absorption and
digestion of fat, vegetables, and meat protein, and the presence of
bacterial or yeast overgrowth. The test sample is stool, or feces, as
the name implies. Below is a list of the parameters tested.[1]

Triglycerides	Chymotrypsin	Meat fibers
Vegetable fibers	Long-chain fatty acids	Cholesterol
Short-chain fatty acids	Bacteria	Yeast/fungi
pH (acidity, alkalinity)		

• *Breath hydrogen/methane test.* Identifies the existence of lactase
deficiency, bacterial overgrowth of the small intestine, or malabsorption.

• *Intestinal permeability test.* See below.

• *Heidelberg gastrogram.* Used by some doctors to measure stomach acidity.

• *Transit time.* The time it takes from when you eat a food to when
it is eliminated as waste (feces) is called the intestinal transit time.
It can be assessed by first taking 200 grains of charcoal tablets with

water (preferably right after a bowel movement) and noting the time of day. Observe the color of your stools over the next 12 to 96 hours (eight days). When you see the first stool that is black, crumbly, and charcoal-looking, record the time and day. The amount of time between taking the tablets and seeing the black stool should be no more than 12 to 18 hours. If it is greater, you should see a health professional who can begin to more specifically address your digestive needs.

Malabsorption and the Leaky Gut Syndrome

The body's normal process of digestion and absorption is designed so that certain substances are absorbed into the bloodstream and other substances are prevented from entering the bloodstream. For example, the vitamins and minerals should be carried across the intestinal wall by a process called active transport, meaning they are helped across by other molecules. Other materials like bacterial fragments or undigested food residue should not be allowed to cross the gut wall.

Malabsorption is a state in which the vitamins, minerals, amino acids, fats, carbohydrates, and other nutrient factors are not properly taken across the intestinal wall into the bloodstream. In the leaky gut syndrome, substances that should not be crossing into the bloodstream are allowed to cross. This often results in an immune response that can lead to a variety of medical problems such as liver disorders, arthritis, fatigue, immune suppression, and more. Ironically, the process by which nutrients are carried across the gut wall is often disrupted as well, so nutrient deficiency may occur. A preliminary study conducted at the Cheney Clinic in collaboration with Great Smokies Diagnostic Laboratory suggests that most people with chronic fatigue syndrome may have increased intestinal permeability.[2]

Laboratory Tests

• *Intestinal permeability test.* There are several ways to measure this, but the most common commercial method involves the consumption of lactulose and mannitol. After several hours you collect a urine sample and the laboratory determines whether reduced or excessive amounts of the sugars have been absorbed.

• *Secretory IgA (sIgA)*. Secretory IgA is an antibody that protects the mucous membrane (lining) of the nose, mouth, lungs, and gut from foreign materials such as viruses, bacteria, food antigens, and chemicals. Some doctors believe low sIgA is an indirect indicator of poor gut defenses and leaky gut. This test is done on a saliva sample.

Treatment

The treatment of malabsorption or leaky gut syndrome is aimed at repairing the damaged intestinal lining, improving digestive enzyme activity, and reducing the load of irritant substances such as drugs, chemicals, and allergens. This is an area of intense interest among clinicians and researchers. More is being discovered each day. Thus, understand that the following list of nutrients will most certainly be revised and improved.

1. *L-Glutamine.* A principal fuel used by the upper GI tract. It prevents the transfer of intestinal bacteria into the body. It is important for the synthesis of antibodies (sIgA) and significantly improves gut immune function. L-Glutamine is essential for maintenance of intestinal mucosal structure, function, and metabolism.[3,4]

2. *Gamma-linolenic acid (GLA).* Derived from evening primrose or borage seed oil, GLA is an important precursor in the formation of an antiinflammatory substance called PGE1. PGE1 helps prevent formation of proinflammatory substances. GLA administered orally is taken up fairly rapidly into intestinal mucosal cells and begins to influence the formation of pro-inflammatory and antiinflammatory compounds.

3. *Butyric acid.* A short-chain fatty acid produced when your beneficial gut bacteria ferment fiber. It is involved in the repair of damaged tissue and hastens regeneration of cells.

4. *Antioxidant nutrients.* Vitamins E and C, beta-carotene, zinc, magnesium, selenium, and glutathione precursors protect against free-radical damage to the intestinal cells.

5. *HCl.* Taken with meals, betaine HCl facilitates digestion in the

stomach, lessening the antigenic load. This is only needed when there is evidence of decreased stomach acidity. It is never used if there is ulceration or intestinal bleeding.

6. *Gamma-oryzanol.* Derived from rice bran oil, this substance has been used to successfully manage inflammatory conditions of the GI tract. In a series of Japanese studies, therapeutic improvement was found to occur in 85 to 90 percent of cases of intestinal disorders ranging from duodenal ulcer to irritable bowel syndrome.[5]

7. *Soluble plant fiber.* This is degraded to short-chain fatty acids such as butyric acid by intestinal microbes. It lowers intestinal permeability and enhances repair of the intestinal lining.

8. *Lactobacillus acidophilus and Bifidobacterium bifidum.* These active cultures reinoculate the bowel with beneficial bacteria.

9. *Bovine antibody complex.* A product known as SpectraPlex is sometimes used to facilitate the elimination of harmful bacteria from the gut and reduce yeast overgrowth. It is available over-the-counter as Inner Strength. Avoid if extremely dairy-sensitive.

10. *N-acetyl-D-glucosamine (NAG).* NAG is a key precursor in the formation of glycoproteins that make up the intestinal lining. This is the most superficial layer and is in contact with gut contents. NAG aids in rebuilding the mucosa, promotes the growth of B. bifidum, and blocks the adherence of some pathogens such as C. albicans to the mucosal surface.[6,7,8]

11. *Ginkgo biloba.* Ginkgo protects the gut lining from free-radical damage.

12. *Plant enzymes and porcine pancreatic enzymes* assist in digestion of protein, fat, and carbohydrate in the small intestine.

13. *Fructooligosaccharides (FOS).* FOS are important growth factors that stimulate the growth of bifidobacteria in the colon.

14. *Adequate water.* Most people consume inadequate amounts of water for optimum health.

15. *Removal of offending foods or food allergens* from the diet.

16. *Avoidance of antiinflammatory drugs* such as aspirin, ibuprofen, and indomethacin. These drugs cause inflammation of the intestinal lining and increased intestinal permeability.

17. *Pantothenic acid.* Aids in cell energy production and repair.

Irritable Bowel Syndrome

Irritable bowel syndrome (IBS) is a chronic gastrointestinal disorder that usually begins in adolescence or early adulthood. I describe it here because chronic fatigue is one of the most common complaints of its sufferers. IBS does have many things in common with our previous discussion, but there are some very specific considerations.

IBS is estimated to affect roughly 30 million American adults or about one-third of the adult population. IBS affects women more than men and commonly runs in families. It is characterized by alternating constipation and diarrhea, which is often accompanied by gas, bloating, cramps, or nausea. Yet this hardly tells the whole story.

Patients who suffer from IBS are plagued by its vague and urgent symptoms, but when they seek diagnosis or treatment find little satisfaction. This is because the colon shows no sign of disease. In the past, this caused doctors to label IBS a disorder of anxious neurotics, but this view is no longer widely held. While there can be certain psychological triggers, irritable bowel syndrome is a real physical malady. The symptoms are not confined to the bowel, as IBS patients often experience irritability in other body systems, especially the muscular system.

People with irritable bowel syndrome tend to have higher rates of chronic tiredness, urinary tract irritation, muscle pain, painful sexual intercourse (women), headache, nausea, difficulty swallowing, bad taste in the mouth, poor sleeping, and several other symptoms. They are also likely to be more sensitive to normal amounts of intestinal gas than people without IBS.

Some of the causes of IBS are discussed below.

Diet. Intolerance to food appears to be a common cause of irritable bowel symptoms. A British study found that certain foods provoked IBS symptoms in roughly two-thirds of patients studied. The most common offenders were wheat, corn, dairy products, coffee, tea, and citrus.[9] Other foods may provoke symptoms in a sensitive individual. It may be wise to be evaluated for food sensitivity. Several recent scientific papers have highlighted this important relationship.[10,11,12,13]

Sugar. Excess sugars can lead to IBS in some people. Included are lactose, fructose, mannitol, glucose, sorbitol, and other sweeteners. Some cause problems in part because they are fermented in the gut and produce gas. Others create problems by causing extra fluid to be absorbed into the bowel, leading to diarrhea. Intolerance to lactose, the sugar in cow's milk, is common in adults. Removal of dairy from the diet has helped many patients with irritable bowel syndrome and fatigue.

Stress. Stress seems to bring on symptoms of IBS in some susceptible individuals.

Bacterial overgrowth. Bacterial overgrowth can occur when antibiotics are used excessively. This occurs, as noted earlier, because beneficial intestinal bacteria can be killed by antibiotics, while nonsusceptible bacteria in the intestines grow out of control.

Yeast overgrowth. Yeast overgrowth, especially of *Candida albicans,* is a negative consequence of antibiotic therapy and can lead to IBS, food intolerance, gas, bloating, fatigue, and many other symptoms.

Lactose intolerance. Many adults do not tolerate the milk sugar lactose and suffer intestinal symptoms whenever milk products are consumed. If you have IBS symptoms, you may wish to consider a three-week period of eliminating all dairy products to see if symptoms improve. One of my former patients, Richard, improved his IBS symptoms simply by removing dairy products from the diet.

Parasites. In 197 patients with IBS, 48 percent tested positive for the parasite Giardia lamblia. Treatment of giardiasis led to improvement of symptoms in roughly 90 percent of the patients studied.[14] This is a surprisingly high percentage. If you have IBS symptoms and haven't found the cause, seriously consider having the appropriate tests run for parasites. See the chapter on hidden infections for tests.

Antibiotic overuse. This can contribute to thinning of intestinal mucosa, translocation of enteric bacteria, overgrowth of pathogens, inflammation, leaky gut, and other intestinal complications. Broad-

spectrum antibiotics are most likely to bring this about, as are prolonged or prophylactic courses.

Antiinflammatory drugs. This is not usually listed as a cause of
IBS. However, doctors are learning more about the adverse effects
on the intestinal lining of drugs like aspirin, ibuprofin, indomethacin,
and other medicines given to relieve pain. If you are on one of these
or a similar drug and suffer from IBS, see your doctor about possibly modifying your prescription.

Signs and Symptoms

> Alternating constipation and diarrhea
> Cramps
> Gas
> Urgency
> Nausea

Various problems associated with IBS and their relative frequency
are summarized below:[15]

Associated Condition	Frequency (%)
Weight loss	65–75
Growth retardation	15–30
Anemia	60–80
Hypergammaglobulinemia	15–40
Iron deficiency	39–81
B_{12} deficiency	>50
Folic acid deficiency	36–54
Minerals (K, Ca, Mg, Zn, Cu, Mn, Mo…)	14–60
Vitamins (A, C, E, B …)	>80

You may have noticed that nutrient deficiency is common in IBS
sufferers. If you suffer from IBS, it is important that a doctor knowledgeable in clinical nutrition make an assessment of your nutritional
status, since such nutrient deficiencies may lead to fatigue as well as
other health problems.

Laboratory Tests

There are no specific laboratory tests for irritable bowel syndrome and there is no truly conclusive test. The diagnosis is made by the presence of defining symptoms and the absence of another disease state. If you have IBS symptoms, especially if they are accompanied by blood in the stool, persistent abdominal pain, or fever, you should see a doctor. Your doctor will likely do some tests to rule out more serious intestinal illness. If your doctor suspects parasites, food intolerance, intestinal dysbiosis, or other problems, he or she will order appropriate tests. Tests to assess intestinal permeability can be revealing.

Treatment

Nutritional biochemist Dr. Jeffrey Bland separates irritable bowel syndrome into three categories, each of which responds to a different approach. His group has found success in approaching IBS in this way.[16]

1. Diarrhea-predominant form:
   a. Usually associated with:
      1) Food intolerance.
      2) Inflammatory substances in the intestinal tract.
      3) Lactose intolerance.
   b. May be helped by:
      1) Eliminating food allergens.
      2) Nutritional supplementation (L-glutamine, zinc, pantothenic acid, EPA, GLA, and others).
      3) Avoidance of known toxins (alcohol, drugs, etc.).
      4) Avoidance of simple sugars.
      5) Adequate dietary fiber.
2. Constipation-predominant form:
   a. Associated with:
      1) Inadequate fiber intake.
      2) Inadequate fluid intake.
      3) Inadequate, irregular exercise.

  b. May be helped by:
    1) Gradually increasing intake of hypoallergenic fiber
     foods.
    2) Increasing fluid intake.
    3) Increasing daily exercise.
    4) Gradually increasing nutrients such as vitamin C and
     magnesium.

 3. Pain/Gas/Bloating-predominant form:
  a. Associated with:
    1) Inadequate secretion of digestive enzymes.
    2) Changes in intestinal bacteria (dysbiosis).
    3) Excess intake of fermentable carbohydrate.

  b. May be helped by:
    1) Elimination fermentable carbohydrate (most grains
     except rice).
    2) Use of digestive aids such as enzymes.
    3) Reinoculation of bowel flora with acidophilus and/or
     bifidus.
    4) Addition of fructooligosaccharides to support
     beneficial bacteria.
    5) Addition of an active bovine milk-derived antibody
     complex (avoid if highly dairy-sensitive).

Ronald had a history of IBS in his family, and suffered himself for twenty years. He had seen numerous different allopathic and holistic doctors, and had made substantial dietary changes over the years. He improved somewhat on the various regimens but continued to be nagged by his symptoms. I suggested he try a product called UltraClear Sustain, developed by Dr. Bland to treat problems of the gastrointestinal lining. After one week on this formula, Ronald noticed dramatic improvement. After three weeks his IBS symptoms had improved by 90 percent. It is difficult to say whether all IBS patients would respond this well to UltraClear Sustain, but Ronald's improvement (and that of many others) was clearly attributable to this formula.

Irritable bowel syndrome can be a complicated disorder to treat. Moreover, there is often overlap among the categories stated above. If you suffer from IBS, it is advisable to see your doctor about tailoring an approach to your specific needs.

In Review

1. Problems of the intestinal tract that affect digestion and absorption can cause fatigue.

2. Disruption of the digestive process at one or more of many stages can impair nutrient assimilation.

3. Altered intestinal permeability, or leaky gut syndrome, often allows material that should not be absorbed into the body to be absorbed. It may also impair the absorption of nutrients.

4. Irritable bowel syndrome affects roughly 30 million Americans or up to one-third of the adult population.

5. The symptoms of IBS are alternating constipation and diarrhea sometimes accompanied by nausea, gas, bloating, or cramping.

6. Food allergens are common contributors to IBS symptoms.

7. Junk food can aggravate IBS symptoms.

8. Management of digestive problems through dietary changes, reduced consumption of allergenic food, and nutritional therapy can often be helpful.

Chapter 3

Food and Fatigue

MANY PEOPLE ARE able to remedy their fatigue by altering their diets in various ways. For example, one of my patients cured her fatigue by stopping all junk food. Another was cured by switching to a vegetarian diet. Another, who had been a vegetarian for many years, improved when she added a small amount of organic meat to her diet every few days. Still another improved by eliminating all dairy products from his diet.

If you suffer from fatigue and haven't considered food as a possible factor, you may have missed something important. Food can influence mood and induce fatigue in at least three basic ways:

1. Food allergic reactions or food intolerance can lead directly or indirectly to fatigue.
2. Refined food, junk foods, and food additives can alter mood, resulting in fatigue. This includes chemical contaminants on food.
3. Certain food combinations affect the mood-altering neurotransmitters in the brain.

Each of these factors is described below.

Food Allergy and Food Intolerance

The idea that intolerance to food adversely influences health is not new. In 1954, Dr. Frederick Speer described the so-called allergic-tension-fatigue syndrome, in which certain foods or food additives were found to provoke symptoms. Among these symptoms were irritability, hyperactivity, insomnia, hypersomnia, impaired concentration, and of course, fatigue.[1] In 1979, Theron Randolph, M.D., pioneering physician and author of *The Alternative Approach to Allergies,* discussed how allergy and intolerance can contribute to fatigue, mental exhaustion, low vitality, depression, confusion, and lethargy.[2] William Philpott, M.D. described the mood-altering effect of food in his book *Brain Allergies* in 1980. In this book he presented the many and varied mood-altering effects that food allergic reactions can trigger.[3]

In talking about adverse reactions to food, we must distinguish between true allergy and intolerance (or hypersensitivity). Allergy exists when a person reacts to a substance as a result of immune-related mechanisms. The term intolerance is used when a person reacts to a substance for other reasons that are not immune system-mediated. An example of true allergy is hay fever, with its itchy eyes, runny nose, and sneezing. An example of intolerance is the temporary sensitivity to food that occurs after a viral or bacterial infection of the intestinal tract. In the latter example, infection alters the permeability of the gut, causing a "leaky gut," which allows undigested food residue to more easily pass into the bloodstream.

Adverse food reactions can elicit almost any symptom and affect almost any body system. Many problems with food allergy or intolerance can be traced to problems within the intestinal tract. Leaky gut syndrome, described earlier, is one contributor to food intolerance. In such cases, food reactions improve when the leaky gut is repaired using nutrients. Food intolerance due to microbial invasion of the intestinal tract is another matter. The yeast *Candida albicans* is a well-known inhabitant of the gut that can contribute to food intolerance. Overgrowth of bacterial organisms such as *Klebsiella pneumoniae* can do likewise. In these instances, substances that eradicate these organisms are helpful, along with alterations in diet and use of probiotics such as acidophilus and bifidus.

Certain foods tend to cause more allergic responses than others. Among the most common offenders are: .

Wheat	Cow's milk/dairy products
Soy	Corn
Peanuts	Eggs

Beyond this list of common offenders, almost any food can provoke a response depending on individual sensitivity.

Derek was a 40-year-old busy professional who loved sports. He complained of chronic fatigue, sore feet, heart palpitations, feelings of anxiety in his chest, occasional headaches, and intestinal upset. When he exercised, which he loved to do, he felt muscle pain and exhaustion for the next two or three days. An IgG food sensitivity assay revealed that he was sensitive to almonds (+1), Egg (+2), peanut (+4), sesame (+2), soybean (+4), and wheat (+2). Reactions denoted +1 are mild, while those denoted +4 are severe, indicating that increased antibodies are present to the offending food. When Derek eliminated these foods from his diet almost all of his symptoms improved.

Interestingly, we later discovered that whenever he consumed wheat his rapid heart beat, heart palpitations, and feelings of anxiety would return. Also of interest was the finding that laboratory assessment showed his antioxidant nutrient status was low, even though he had been taking antioxidants. Once he removed the offending foods from his diet his antioxidant levels eventually increased. My interpretation of this finding is that adverse food reactions can cause inflammation of the intestinal lining and contribute to poor nutrient uptake. When offending substances are removed, nutrient uptake often improves.

Laboratory Tests

A number of different tests are used to assess allergic sensitivity or intolerance to food. This can be done in three basic ways: blood tests, skin tests, or food-elimination tests.

- IgG food sensitivity assay
- IgE RAST
- Elimination/Provocation
- Intradermal cutaneous test
- Scratch test

Allergists commonly perform scratch tests of the skin, but this is not always accurate in identifying allergy or intolerance to food. Another skin test in common use is the intradermal cutaneous test, in which a small amount of a suspected offender is injected just beneath the surface of the skin. The doctor observes the area for a characteristic reaction.

Because of the limitations of skin tests, many doctors use blood tests to assess allergic sensitivity. Blood tests in use today include tests for antibodies designated IgE, IgA, IgG, and IgM. These tests look for proteins produced by the immune system in response to offending substances.

The most commonly used test to detect immediate reactions is called an IgE RAST (radioallergosorbent test). These types of reactions, called immediate hypersensitivity reactions, classically involve symptoms such as itchy eyes, runny nose, wheezing, hives, difficulty swallowing, and difficulty breathing. The reaction often comes on within minutes to hours of eating the offending food. IgE RAST tests are helpful but do not detect the late-phase or delayed-onset reactions that may take hours to days to manifest.

The IgG food sensitivity assay is helpful in detecting a particular kind of delayed-onset allergic reaction. It is a useful screening test, especially in those who have not been on food avoidance programs. The ELISA/ACT is another test that measures delayed sensitivity reactions to food. This test also measures reactivity to chemicals and additives.

One of the most widely accepted forms of testing is the elimination-provocation test. With this method, one is first placed on a diet that excludes foods that commonly trigger allergic reactions. The diet is continued for one to four weeks. After this time, suspected foods are added back to the diet one at a time. If any food produces symptoms upon reintroduction, the food is deemed an offender and must be avoided. Elimination/provocation is still considered the "gold standard" among allergy tests. Its main limitation is that it requires time, effort and compliance on the part of the patient.

Junk Food, Food Additives, and Chemicals

Junk food consumption can also be a factor in fatigue. Richard is a classic example. At age 39, he "just felt tired all the time" and "never felt alert and refreshed." He vowed to eliminate all sources of refined sugar. After three weeks of going relatively "sugar-free" his energy improved substantially. He no longer experiences fatigue as he once did.

Junk food, which includes almost any processed food, is generally low in essential nutrients. Consumption of processed foods as a significant portion of the diet eventually leads to essential nutrient insufficiency. In chapter 4, I describe the common finding of magnesium deficiency in patients with chronic fatigue and low vitality. Consumption of certain types of junk food may precipitate magnesium loss. Soda pop is a good example. Cola-type beverages are buffered with phosphoric acid. Phosphoric acid consumption can cause increased amounts of magnesium to be lost through the urine. It has been shown that when a person consumes a 12-ounce can of cola, he or she may lose up to 36 milligrams of magnesium through the urine. To put this in perspective, the average American consumes 365 servings of soda pop each year. The average 12- to 29-year-old consumes 638 cans per year.[4]

Mary was a commodities trader in the Minneapolis area. She worked long, stressful hours in a highly volatile, rapidly changing field. She ate poorly and had many physical complaints. Her most pressing complaint was fatigue, since she was becoming less able to function to her normal capacity. She also had cardiac arrhythmia, severe headaches, and blood pressure problems. I made many recommendations to Mary, but her willingness to make great changes was simply not there.

In the initial examination she told me she consumed about 12 cans of Pepsi each day. I felt that if she would at least cut out the pop she would experience some improvement that might encourage her to make other changes. She was willing to eliminate the Pepsi, but asked me with some consternation, "What will I drink?" I replied with incredulity, "Why, water, of course." It seemed like a foreign substance to Mary.

Mary eliminated all pop from her diet. Her change in energy and decrease in headache symptoms was almost immediate. Her arrhythmia also improved, which is not surprising given the function of magnesium in heart muscle. Eventually most of her fatigue symptoms improved, but her magnesium status, while much better, had not returned to normal. I placed her on a magnesium supplement and she fully recovered. An interesting side note to this story is that Mary had been unsuccessful at conceiving a child for several years. After eliminating pop and restoring her magnesium levels to normal, she finally conceived and gave birth to a little boy.

I am frequently asked if there really is a difference between a "fortified" processed food diet and a whole foods diet. The answer is always "yes." The question that usually follows is "Are organic whole foods more nutritious than commercially grown whole foods?" I have believed for many years that organic foods are more nutritious based on what I saw with patients. Some recent research seems to give credence to that observation.

Bob Smith, director of Doctor's Data medical laboratory in Chicago, published the results of a study he conducted comparing the mineral content of organic foods versus commercially grown supermarket foods. The foods analyzed by his laboratory included apples, pears, potatoes, wheat, and sweet corn. He did not measure the ash value as many previous studies have done, but the "wet" value as one would encounter the food in a supermarket or food co-op. Smith found that organic pears, apples, potatoes, and wheat had, on an average, over 90 percent more of the nutritional elements than similar commercial food, and if sweet corn levels are included, the average difference is more than two and one half times.[5]

Average: Organic vs. Commercial

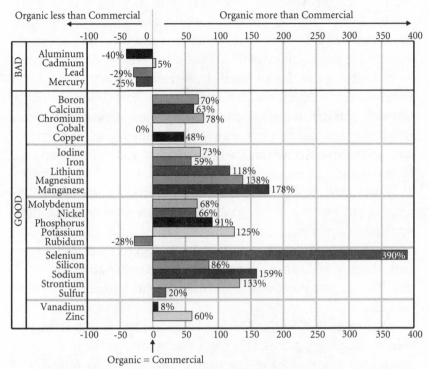

Organic less than Commercial ← | → Organic more than Commercial

Organic = Commercial

Reproduced with permission. *J. Appl. Nutr.* (1993; 45(1):35–39)

An added advantage of organic foods is they have lower levels of pesticide and herbicide residues. In a summary of pesticide and herbicide levels in food published in *Pesticide Alert* by Mott and Snyder, many foods were shown to contain detectable biocide residues above the safety limit. For example, high biocide levels were found on 86 percent of domestic strawberries, on 78 percent of cantaloupe, and on 70 percent of tomatoes.[6] When you realize that the "safe limit" is arbitrarily set, that many biocides have unknown effects on the body, and that many biocides are not even tested, the picture looks very unfriendly indeed. Given the high nutrient value of organic food and the chemical contaminants of some commercial foods, the choice of certified organic food (especially if you are in poor health) seems wise.

Food additives may also cause symptoms of fatigue. The more notable ones are listed below.

Aspartame (NutraSweet™) is number one on the list of complaints to the FDA, accounting for roughly 85 percent of all complaints. It is currently found in more than 3,000 foods. The main components of aspartame are L-phenylalanine (50 percent), L-aspartic acid (40 percent), and methanol (wood alcohol, 10 percent). Once in the body, the methanol can be converted into formaldehyde via a well-documented chemical reaction. Aspartic acid is an excitatory neurotransmitter that is toxic to the nervous system at high levels. Headache, fatigue, and irritability are among the most common symptoms reported to occur, with aspartame soft drinks being the most common source.

A 1993 article in *Biological Psychiatry* points out some of the concerns about aspartame, especially in people with mood disorders. Forty patients with depression were to be given aspartame or placebo for seven days. Those on aspartame experienced such severe reactions that the Institutional Review Board of the hospital demanded the study be terminated after only 13 patients had completed the trial.[7]

Aspartame has been called an excitotoxin by some neuroscientists because the aspartic acid component mimics the body's natural excitatory system in the brain. This system is now under suspicion of contributing to a variety of neurological disorders. Neurologists such as Dr. Russell Blaylock have begun to sound the alarm about aspartame's ability to trigger neurological damage. In his book, *Excitotoxins*, Blaylock cites many studies in humans and animals showing the cumulative affects of aspartame on the brain. He further shows that the affects of aspartame are increased when brain energy pathways are sluggish or when levels of certain nutrients such as magnesium, DHA, or vitamin E are low. This is precisely the state of affairs in many fatigued patients. Thus, fatigued patients should avoid additives like aspartame where possible.

Sulfites are second only to aspartame in generating complaints to the FDA. Sulfites are bleaching agents used in processed foods, dried fruits, packaged potato products, drugs, wine, and many other foods. They produce hypersensitivity reactions that can be severe. Asthmatics appear to be most susceptible. Some patients who do not tolerate sulfites may have an enzyme deficiency that responds to vitamin B_{12}, folic acid, and molybdenum.

BHT/BHA are preservatives found in many processed foods. They may provoke symptoms of headache and behavior changes in sensitive individuals.

MSG is a flavor enhancer that is also known excitotoxin to the brain. In excess, it appears to activate a receptor in the brain that causes excess calcium to flood into brain cells causing them to swell and malfunction. If too severe, the brain cells may die. The harmful affects of MSG on the brain appear to be amplified when there is poor brain energy, a person has not eaten enough, the person is under stress, or the person is deficient in one or more of some 15 different nutrients.

Coffee and caffeine. The key fatigue-inducing ingredient in coffee is caffeine. Caffeine is also found in many prescription drugs as well as in soda pop. It may seem odd that the stimulant caffeine can cause fatigue, but it can. There are two primary ways in which caffeine seems to cause fatigue: by overstimulating the body and nervous system and by interfering with the amount and quality of sleep. In my experience, many fatigued patients who either eliminate or reduce their caffeine consumption have a noticeable improvement in energy. Some who go off caffeine experience significant withdrawal symptoms. If you are one of these, chances are that caffeine is contributing to your fatigue.

Alcohol. Alcohol contributes to nutrient loss and thus poor nutritional status, changes in sleep habits, kidney and liver distress, brain and memory impairment, and numerous other problems. Each of these is associated with symptoms of fatigue and low energy. Alcohol can damage the intestinal lining and lead to leaky gut syndrome and is a well-known cause of thiamin deficiency. If you consume alcohol on a regular basis, it may be a source of your fatigue. Fatigue is a consistent manifestation of alcoholism.

Sugar. Excess sugar consumption is an important cause of fatigue. This is especially true of those who suffer from hypoglycemia, or low blood sugar. Many patients have experienced vastly improved energy by merely eliminating this one "antinutrient."

Food Combinations and Mood

There is a most interesting relationship between your choice of food and your mood. It is based primarily on how your body converts certain food constituents and how they are delivered to the brain. While there are many neurochemicals that influence the brain and mood, there are two of primary interest. Both are directly affected by dietary choices. These neurochemicals are tryptophan and tyrosine, both amino acids (recall the building blocks of protein). Tryptophan is converted into the neurotransmitter serotonin, which is calming, relaxing, and can be sleep-inducing. Tyrosine is converted into the neurotransmitters dopamine and norepinephrine, which stimulate alertness. According to researcher Judith Wurtman, Ph.D., by choosing the wrong combinations of protein, fat, and carbohydrate, you might be alert when you want to be relaxed or sleepy when you want to be alert.[8]

Carbohydrates fall into two basic categories: simple and complex. Simple carbohydrates include things like sucrose from table sugar. Complex carbohydrates, often referred to as starches, are found in foods like potatoes. Both simple and complex carbohydrates trigger the release of insulin, which assists in transfer of tryptophan into the brain. This leads to production of more serotonin, a more calm and relaxed state, and possible sluggishness. Therefore, a diet that consists primarily of carbohydrate is more likely to cause fatigue and tiredness.

For example, in 1989 a paper was published in the *Journal of Clinical Psychiatry* reporting on a study of women who fasted overnight, ate a standard breakfast, and at lunch consumed a high-carbohydrate, low-protein meal. They compared these results to those of women eating a meal with relatively similar amounts of protein and carbohydrate (according to established ratios) and those consuming a high-protein, low-carbohydrate meal. Only the high-carbohydrate meal significantly caused fatigue. (It was not related to hypoglycemia.) According to the researchers, fatigue began as soon as the meal elevated the blood levels of tryptophan.[9]

Foods high in simple sugars include doughnuts, pastries, cookies, pie, soft drinks, cake, candy, jellies, and syrup.[10] Foods high in complex carbohydrates include bread, crackers, muffins, potatoes, pasta, rice, barley, corn, kasha, oatmeal and other cereals (unless milk is added, which contains enough protein to inhibit the production of serotonin; however, if you are milk-sensitive this can make you fatigued).

High-fat food can also produce sluggishness and fatigue. When you consume a meal high in fat the digestive process takes longer, which requires that more blood be diverted to the stomach and intestines. This results in less blood being sent to the brain. The symptoms include fatigue, mental dullness, drowsiness, and lethargy. If this type of meal is a regular part of your culinary experience, a chronic sense of fatigue and sluggishness is likely to be the price.

High fat foods include beef (unless lean), whole cow's milk, ice cream, hard cheeses, butter, mayonnaise, creamed soups, creamed vegetables, gravies, lunch meats, organ meats, lamb, and pork products.[11]

Fruit and vegetables will not produce the relaxed, sluggish, fatigued response since they do not have the same effect on production of neurotransmitters.

In summary, if you eat carbohydrate alone, without protein, more tryptophan will be available to the brain and more serotonin will be made. You will feel more relaxed, less anxious, and perhaps more sluggish. This may be desirable before bedtime, but not in mid-afternoon. If you eat protein alone or with a carbohydrate, the brain will likely make more dopamine and norepinephrine. You will be more alert, energetic, and less fatigued. If you eat a meal high in fat, digestion will proceed more slowly, the brain will receive less blood, and you will feel more sluggish.

Eating Right for Optimum Energy

If you go to your local bookstore or health food store you will encounter an unbelievable array of books related to "the right diet." This might include a diet for arthritis, multiple sclerosis, diabetes, weight loss, irritable bowel syndrome, heart disease, a better sex life, and on and on. Some of the books are on target, some are not.

How does the average person make any sense of this? To be honest, I'm not sure how you do, because it often takes a great deal of knowledge of nutrition and metabolism to figure out whether the author's claims make sense and whether the research is sound. Most lay people are not equipped to do this.

Making this task more difficult is the fact that many of the so-called authorities disagree about some of the most fundamental concepts. This is because there is no single diet strategy that suits everyone. Each person is unique biochemically, physically, and emotionally. The diet that suits a tall, thin, small-boned man is not likely the optimum diet for a large-boned, short, 200-pound woman. The Dean Ornish program for reversing heart disease requires that one eat less than 10 percent of their calories as fat. This is excellent for the person with coronary artery blockage but would be disaster for the endurance athlete, since more fat and more calories are needed.

Even though there is no diet that fits everyone, some basic suggestions can be made.

1. Make sure you get enough calories. For the average adult man or woman that means at least 2,000 calories a day—more if you are physically active.

2. Eat five or six small meals each day. Spreading the meals out over the day regulates blood sugar more evenly and puts less stress on the digestive tract.

3. Minimize or eliminate refined food or processed food. Even though some may be fortified with a few token nutrients, these foods are nutrient-poor, contain antinutrients, and will gradually lead you to a nutrient-insufficient state. Many of the byproducts of processing contribute to degenerative diseases.

4. Limit or avoid food additives such as aspartame, MSG, BHT, and others. Many require nutrients in order to be metabolized and eliminated from the body. Some have direct neurotoxic and immunotoxic effects.

5. If you consume meat, consider organic or range-fed meat. These have been raised free of hormones, antibiotics, and other chemicals and do not contribute as heavily to the toxic load. They also tend to be leaner.

6. Try to obtain regionally grown produce where possible. Imported produce is often treated with agricultural chemicals banned in the United States.

7. Use organic produce where possible. Higher nutrient content and lower pesticide residues are good reasons.

8. As a general rule of thumb, attempt to balance your food intake with the following amounts:
   - 65 percent carbohydrate
   - 20 percent protein
   - 15–20 percent fat

9. Consume six to eight eight-ounce glasses of pure water each day. Juice, tea, and coffee don't count. Water is necessary to detoxify and eliminate metabolic waste products and environmental chemicals, not to mention its importance in routine body functions.

10. Exercise regularly. It may seem odd to include exercise along with dietary recommendations, but without exercise you do not burn fat as efficiently and may not regulate blood sugar as efficiently.

A thorough discussion of diets to fit individual needs is found in *Healing with Whole Foods* by Paul Pitchford, North Atlantic Books, Berkeley, California.

In Review

1. Food is an important contributor to fatigue. Food-related factors should be among the first things you consider if you suffer from fatigue, low vitality, or lack of energy.

2. Food-related problems fall into three basic areas: 1) Food allergy or food intolerance, 2) consumption of high-calorie low-nutrient junk food, and 3) food combinations that affect mood by virtue of brain chemicals that are manufactured.

Chapter 4

Vitamins, Minerals, and Fatigue

As YOU READ this chapter, remember our discussion from chapter 1 about energy production. Without adequate vitamins, minerals, amino acids, essential fatty acids, and other essential substances, the production of energy in the human body does not occur efficiently. The nutrients described in this chapter (that are helpful in people with chronic fatigue) are not obscure. They are commonly insufficient or deficient in people in the U.S., Europe, and other nations with similar lifestyles.

This chapter describes a number of nutrients that when present in insufficient amounts can contribute to fatigue and low vitality. Under each nutrient are listed the signs and symptoms that can occur with insufficiency or deficiency of that nutrient. Keep in mind that not all the signs and symptoms need be present in order for that nutrient deficiency to be suspected.

Before we begin, I want you to understand a key distinction between insufficiency and deficiency. The term **deficiency** usually refers to a state in which inadequate amounts of a nutrient lead to a particular disease state or fall outside of a predetermined laboratory reference range. **Insufficiency** refers to a condition in which inadequate amounts of a nutrient are available to allow the body to function at its peak. In the progression from health to disease we commonly pass through phases where insufficiency first develops, followed by deficiency, and then disease. Symptoms can occur at any stage.

Health $\rightarrow$ Insufficiency $\rightarrow$ Deficiency $\rightarrow$ Disease

Vitamin C is a good example. The National Academy of Sciences has set the RDA (recommended daily allowance) for vitamin C at 60 mg per day. This, they say, is more than enough to prevent the *deficiency* disease scurvy. However, many aspects of health can suffer before one develops scurvy. Studies at the USDA found that the activity of white blood cells is directly related to the dietary amounts of vitamin C. At 500 mg (almost ten times the RDA) white blood cells are highly active. At 250 mg their activity declines substantially. At the RDA level their activity is sluggish.[1] During active infection, the body may require 1,000 to 6,000 mg of vitamin C just to maintain white blood cell activity at its normal level.[2]

Other studies have shown that vitamin C is critical for our detoxication of environmental chemicals to which we might be exposed. Since all of us are exposed to at least low levels of pollutants, it would make sense to have adequate amounts of vitamin C in our tissues. Sixty milligrams of vitamin C might be enough to prevent scurvy, but it is *insufficient* to optimize your immune function and protect you from harmful chemicals.

Dr. John Pangborn, of Bionostics, Inc. in Chicago, has reviewed the laboratory results of several thousand cases submitted to him from doctors throughout North America. He has observed that roughly two-thirds of chronic fatigue patients were fatigued as a result of an essential nutrient deficiency.[3] Paul Cheney, M.D., a leading chronic fatigue researcher, has pointed out that chronic fatigue is likely a disorder of energy metabolism, which is a process that requires multiple enzymes. Cheney suggests that stimulating the enzymes of energy production using nutrients such as B-vitamins, magnesium, and CoQ_{10} at above-RDA levels is critical to improving energy production.[4]

With this in mind, we can move forward and discuss the most common nutrient insufficiencies and deficiencies associated with fatigue.

Amino Acids

As mentioned earlier, amino acids are the building blocks of proteins, enzymes, and neurohormones, and they serve as a source of energy for many bodily processes. There are eight essential amino acids that must be derived from the diet. There are 22 main amino acids used in the formation of the body's proteins, 14 of which the body can make if it has the eight essential amino acids. Aside from this there are dozens of other amino acid intermediates in the body.

When an imbalance in amino acid metabolism occurs, it is called an amino acidopathy. This can occur as a result of a vitamin or mineral deficiency since both are important in modifying amino acids for various body functions. For example, magnesium is necessary for the conversion of the amino acid methionine to cysteine. If magnesium is insufficient, you can become deficient in cysteine, which leads to functional changes in your body. Conversion of the amino acid tyrosine to the neurotransmitter epinephrine is vitamin B_6-dependent. Insufficient B_6, which is somewhat common, leads to changes in the production of brain chemicals.

Alexander Bralley, Ph.D., director of MetaMetrix Medical Research Laboratory in Norcross, Georgia, conducted a study of 25 patients with chronic fatigue syndrome. He and his colleagues analyzed the amino acids of each person and found deficiency to be common. The most notable deficiencies included (in order of frequency) tryptophan, phenylalanine, taurine, isoleucine, and leucine. The other deficiencies were not as common. Bralley's group then supplemented each person with vitamin B_6, the eight essential amino acids, and the amino acids that were deficient. After a three-month period of supplementation, near complete improvement in symptoms was seen in 75 percent of the people.[5]

According to John Pangborn, Ph.D., there are two major types of problems related to amino acid imbalance and a third category that occurs less frequently.[6]

1. *Deficiency or insufficiency of one or more of the eight essential amino acids* (more than one is common). Deficiency is

usually due to intestinal malabsorption, which occurs because of one or more of the following:

- insufficient stomach acid
- inflammation of the small intestine
- food allergies (which can cause intestinal inflammation)
- deficiency of pancreatic enzymes (which normally reduce proteins into amino acids)
- poor pancreas function

The eight essential amino acids are:

Isoleucine	Leucine
Lysine	Methionine
Phenylalanine	Threonine
Tryptophan	Valine

2. *Vitamin B_6 deficiency.* Vitamin B_6 is a cofactor in amino acid metabolism. When B_6 levels are inadequate it can lead to abnormal levels of one or more of 14 different amino acids.

3. *Chemical exposure,* which prevents the kidneys from retaining amino acids and can lower essential nutrients.

Signs and Symptoms

The most common symptoms of amino acidopathies include vague tiredness, weakness, body aches, digestive problems, inability to concentrate, and many of the symptoms of food allergy and chemical sensitivity. Because of the role of amino acids in protein formation, enzyme activity, immune function, brain function, liver function, energy production, and countless other processes, amino acid deficiency can contribute to symptoms that affect almost any body system.

Laboratory Tests

- 24-hour urine amino acid analysis
- Plasma amino acid analysis

Supplementation

Supplementation with amino acids can be a tricky matter. It is important to know which amino acids are actually deficient, which are altered because of co-factor deficiency (such as B_{12} or B_6), and which imbalances might be due to poor absorption and digestion. A blood or urine test is the best way to determine these things. Supplementation is best carried out after a knowledgeable health professional has determined your amino acid status.

Foods high in vitamin B_6 include cabbage, cauliflower, avocados, whole grains, bananas, meats, soybeans, egg yolk, fish, dried beans, and peanuts.

L-Carnitine

L-carnitine is an amino acid that deserves special attention because of its important role in the production of energy and its value in helping people with fatigue. L-carnitine is not one of the 22 protein amino acids. It has a highly specialized function. L-carnitine is responsible for carrying fatty acids (the fuel) across the membrane of the mitochondria. Recall that mitochondria are the tiny, power-packed, energy-producing structures inside cells. They are like the furnace where the fuel is burned. When carnitine levels are inadequate, fatty acids are not properly brought into the mitochondria and energy is not efficiently produced. When more carnitine is available, fatty acids are more quickly converted into energy (ATP) and are less likely to be stored as fat.

Carnitine is highest in heart muscle, with most of its vital functions being carried out there. Brain and muscle also contain significant amounts of carnitine. Carnitine has been helpful to people with chronic fatigue, elevated blood fats, poor circulation, certain cardiac problems, neurological disorders, muscle disorders, obesity, and other problems. Carnitine is often given with coenzyme Q_{10}, since CoQ_{10} helps in the intermediate steps of energy production within the mitochondria.

A 1994 study published in *Clinical Infectious Diseases* found that people with chronic fatigue syndrome had considerably lower blood carnitine level than 308 healthy subjects (whose carnitine levels were normal). Improvement in energy was associated with normalization of blood carnitine levels. The researchers suggested that measuring carnitine in blood could be very helpful in people with fatigue.[7]

Carnitine is found primarily in meat (thus the name *carnitine*) and in trace amounts in other foods. It is, therefore, sometimes deficient in vegetarians. It is commonly deficient in those with heart disease, elevated blood fats, obesity, liver disease, energy problems such as fatigue, and in athletes who train heavily.

Signs and Symptoms

The signs of carnitine deficiency or insufficiency have not been clearly defined. Conditions in which carnitine insufficiency might be suspected include:

Elevated blood fats   Fatigue and low vitality
Cardiovascular symptoms   Muscle weakness

Laboratory Tests

Though believed to be somewhat common, carnitine deficiency is difficult to detect. This is because carnitine is higher in tissues like the heart, brain, liver, and muscle, from which it is hard to get a sample. Urine and blood levels do not directly reflect the levels in body tissues. Available tests include:

• Plasma carnitine (a fair reflection of muscle carnitine)[8]

• Red cell carnitine (does not reflect muscle carnitine)

• Muscle carnitine (most accurate but requires a muscle biopsy)

Supplementation

Carnitine is often given therapeutically, based on the illness pattern and its history of success in treating certain disorders. It is usually given in doses of 1,000 to 2,000 mg per day. L-carnitine should be the only form taken. D-carnitine can be toxic and should not be consumed.

Coenzyme Q_{10}

Coenzyme Q_{10}, also known as ubiquinone, is an essential substance required by all cells for energy production. It is an integral part of the energy pathways in mitochondria, which are responsible for generating about 95 percent of the total energy needed by the body. The ultimate product of CoQ_{10} metabolism is ATP. CoQ_{10} is found in body tissues that have a high energy requirement such as heart, muscle, immune cells, and liver. CoQ_{10} is a potent antioxidant, much like vitamin E. Therefore, it is important in protecting the cells against free-radical damage. It may be especially important in protecting LDL cholesterol from damage.

When CoQ_{10} is deficient, organs cannot meet their essential energy requirements. In such cases, supplementation is vitally important.

Many doctors who work with fatigued patients find that CoQ_{10} supplementation is very helpful. In their book *Chronic Fatigue Self-Care Manual*, Paul Cheney and Charles Lapp state that CoQ_{10} is "particularly useful for improving fatigue, thought processes, muscular function, and cardiac complaints. A threshold effect occurs and it may take 5 to 6 weeks for full benefit."[9]

Signs and Symptoms

The signs and symptoms of coenzyme Q_{10} insufficiency have not been clearly established. One might suspect insufficiency in the following circumstances:[10]

Chronic fatigue	Immune insufficiency or
Heavy exercise	recurrent infections
Elevated LDL	Heart abnormalities
Hypertension	Gum disease (gingivitis)

Laboratory Tests

• Serum coenzyme Q_{10}

Supplementation

CoQ_{10} is commonly given in doses ranging from 30 to 200 mg daily for up to six weeks. If energy improvement is noted in this time, supplementation is usually continued. CoQ_{10} levels are highest in beef, chicken, lamb, turkey, and eggs. Plants such as spinach, alfalfa, potato, wheat, and soybean contain CoQ_{10}, but in much lower amounts.

Essential Fatty Acids

Essential fatty acids (EFAs) are long-chain unsaturated fats that must be obtained from the diet. The two main categories of unsaturated fatty acids are designated omega-6 and omega-3. Omega-6 fatty acids are most common in foods like sunflower and corn oil. Omega-3 fatty acids are high in flax oil and fish oil. Each of these families of fatty acids have important roles to play in 1) the production of energy, 2) the formation of prostaglandins, which among other things regulate inflammation, immune function, circulation, and other body functions, and 3) the formation of the membranes of body cells. Without adequate dietary essential fatty acids these processes begin to falter and poor health results.

In 1990, researchers from Scotland and Canada reported on their study of essential fatty acid supplementation in 63 patients with postviral fatigue syndrome (PVFS), exhaustion, weakness, poor concentration, and other symptoms common to PVFS. In the fatigued patients, red cell levels of omega-3 and omega-6 fatty acids were well below normal. Each was then given a supplement containing 80 percent evening primrose oil (a rich source of gamma-linolenic acid [GLA]) and 20 percent concentrated fish oil (a rich source of eicosapentaenoic acid [EPA] and docosahexaenoic acid [DHA]). EFA supplementation caused improvement in 74 percent of patients after one month and 85 percent after three months (23 and 17 percent respectively for placebo group). Not only did symptoms improve, but red cell fatty acid levels returned to normal.[11]

Essential fatty acids require a number of co-factors in order to be properly converted into their active states. These include magnesium, B_6, B_3, iron, zinc, vitamin C, folic acid, and biotin. Supplementation with these factors generally enhances the effectiveness of fatty acid therapy.

When EFAs are heated, hydrogenated, exposed to air, or processed in some other way, they undergo a dramatic structural change. They convert from the normal cis-form, which is U-shaped to what's called a trans-form, which is more arrow-shaped. This change causes the fatty acid to be unusable for many of its normal metabolic functions. When trans-fatty acids are incorporated into cell membranes in your body, their presence makes the cell more rigid and inflexible—not a healthy situation. In fact, trans-fatty acids are *solid* at body temperature, not fluid like the normal cis-fatty acids. Trans-fatty acids set the stage for inflammation and have been implicated in heart disease, inflammatory illness, autoimmune disorders, immune deficiency, skin problems, and numerous other conditions.

One of the main problems with trans-fatty acids is that they antagonize the good, or cis-, fatty acids. Trans-fatty acids are present in high amounts in the diets of most people in the United States. Common foods include french fries, chicken nuggets, deep-fried fish burgers, chips, pastries, cookies, candies, cakes, and margarine. In fact, margarine has some of the highest concentrations of trans-fatty acids of any food and has even been banned in the Netherlands because of this.

Below is a list of common foods and the percent of fat that occurs as trans-fatty acids. You should reduce your consumption of trans-fatty acids at every opportunity. They contribute to a tremendous variety of health problems, including poor energy.[12,13,14]

Signs and Symptoms

Dandruff	Dry scalp
Dry, unmanageable hair	Brittle, easily frayed nails
"Alligator skin"	Patches of pale skin on cheeks
Abnormal ear wax	Allergies
Excessive thirst	Eczema
Poor wound healing	Infections
Weakness	Fatigue

Follicular hyperkeratosis ("chicken skin" on backs of arms)

The Trans Fatty Acid Content of Common Food

Food Source	% of Fat as Trans Fatty Acids*
Breads and Rolls	1.8–24
Cakes and cookies	30–40
Candy and Frostings	38.6
Crackers	20–30
French Fries	37.4
Margarine	
Hard	6–47.8
Soft	6–17
Pastries	33.5
Vegetable Shortening	37.3
Corn Chips	24–30

J. Am. Oil Chem. Soc., 1983; 60: 1788–95.
Nut. Rev., 1984; 42(8)

*Less than 1 or 2 percent trans fatty acids is ideal.

Laboratory Tests

Many doctors give essential fatty acids based on symptoms, history, and their clinical judgment without resorting to blood tests. This is reasonable since EFAs are quite safe and effective, and only recently have accurate tests for EFAs become commercially available. However, blood tests for EFAs can be extremely revealing. They show the levels of various EFAs and their metabolites. You can get an indication of whether blocks are occurring in fatty acid conversion or if dietary deficiencies exist. An additional test shows to what extent fatty acids are being damaged, or oxidized. The tests most often used include:

• Red cell fatty acid analysis

• Plasma fatty acid analysis

• Total lipid peroxides

• Thiobarbituric acid reactive substances (TBARS)

Supplementation

Essential fatty acids are widely available in supplemental form. GLA is obtained from primrose oil, borage oil, or black currant seed oil. EPA and DHA are obtained from fish oil. LNA, or linolenic acid, is obtained from flax oil. Essential fatty acids are easily destroyed by cooking, heat, light, and oxygen. Therefore, they should always be refrigerated and should never be used for cooking. If you have stored them opened for more than a few months, they are likely rancid and must be discarded. This is especially true of flax oil since it is usually sold in liquid form and not perles. Whenever essential fatty acids are taken, additional vitamin E must be taken or oxidation to the delicate EFAs can more easily occur.

Folic Acid

Folic acid is a vitamin that is widely available in food, but it is easily destroyed by cooking and storage. Up to 100 percent of the vitamin can be destroyed if food is overcooked or improperly stored. If few fresh foods are consumed, especially green leafy vegetables, folic acid easily becomes deficient. A diet high in milk, eggs, meats, fruits, and root vegetables such as potatoes would be low in folic acid. A diet containing fresh green leafy vegetables, broccoli, asparagus, kidney beans, and whole-grain bread would be considered high in folic acid. According to a 1989 study, the daily intake of folic acid for adults between the ages of 19 and 74 was roughly 242 micrograms.[15] This is far lower than the conservative RDA of 400 mcg per day.

Folic acid is necessary for the manufacture of blood cells and for various other metabolic processes. Deficiency of folic acid can lead to a condition known as megaloblastic anemia, which is associated with fatigue. However, fatigue can be associated with insufficiency of folic acid before anemia develops.

Folic acid needs double during pregnancy. Supplementation with folic acid is advised for all women during pregnancy to prevent neural tube defects. Supplementation may also be helpful to remedy some of the fatigue that comes with pregnancy.

Folic acid deficiency is one of the most common vitamin deficiencies of all and is the most common nutritional deficiency of the elderly. Folic acid deficiency occurs in five to thirty percent of people over 65. Numerous prescription drugs commonly used by the elderly can contribute to folic acid deficiency, such as Dilantin, phenobarbital, cholestyramine, and aspirin. Those over 65 also commonly consume a diet that is low in folic acid. About 35 percent of people with chemical sensitivity have low blood folic acid.[16]

Signs and Symptoms

The signs and symptoms are almost indistinguishable from those of B_{12} deficiency.

Fatigue	Irritability
Weakness	Loss of appetite
Shortness of breath	Sore tongue or mouth
Forgetfulness	Intestinal disturbance

Laboratory Tests

- Formiminoglutamic acid
- Urinary homocystine (barring B_{12} or B_6 deficiency)
- Red cell folic acid
- Serum folic acid

Supplementation

A folic acid supplement is usually given by mouth. Four hundred to 1,000 mcg daily is a common dose. One caveat is in order. Folic acid supplementation can improve the blood cell findings as well as relieve symptoms of fatigue. However, if folic acid is given to someone who is B_{12}-deficient and B_{12} is not given, the neurological signs of B_{12} deficiency can be masked and become worse. Thus, high levels of folic acid should not be taken unless B_{12} deficiency has been ruled out. Also, folic acid supplementation should be avoided in people with high blood histamine.

Glutathione

Glutathione is a compound made of the amino acids cysteine, glycine, and glutamic acid. It is a potent antioxidant substance and important in detoxification of foreign chemicals and toxic minerals. Glutathione protects muscle tissue from damage during heavy exercise, during which glutathione stores drop substantially. Body glutathione levels appear to decline with age. In fact, whole blood glutathione levels are being used as an index of human aging.[17,18]

The trace element selenium is an important cofactor with glutathione because of its role in the enzyme glutathione peroxidase. This substance is needed to detoxify peroxides that are generated during many bodily functions.

The four primary functions of glutathione include:

• Antioxidant activity

• Detoxification of toxic chemicals and heavy metals

• Lymphocyte formation and other aspects of immune function

• Protecting the integrity of red blood cells

A recent report in the *Archives of Environmental Health* illustrates the importance of glutathione in detoxication and protection from toxic substances. Firefighters had been exposed to polychlorinated biphenyls (PCBs) while fighting an electrical fire. Many came down with symptoms consistent with chronic fatigue syndrome and others with multiple chemical sensitivity. Those who were exposed but did not become ill tended to have higher blood levels of glutathione. When a detoxification program was initiated that included supplemental glutathione, those with health complaints improved in overall health.[19]

Signs and Symptoms

The signs of glutathione deficiency have not been established. Circumstances in which glutathione insufficiency might be suspected include:

Chronic fatigue	Burns or trauma
Infectious diseases	Chemical exposure
Multiple chemical sensitivity	Heavy exercise
Intestinal malabsorption	Parasitic infection
Cysteine deficiency	Vegetarianism with low protein intake

Laboratory Tests

• Whole blood glutathione

Supplementation

The most common substances used to improve glutathione levels are cysteine, N-acetylcysteine, and reduced L-glutathione. Some have suggested that glutathione taken by mouth is broken down in the gut and not absorbed. However, glutathione has a specific form of amino acid linkage that is not broken down by digestive enzymes. Anyone on N-acetylcysteine may need to take additional copper or zinc, since NAC may bind these nutrients when used for prolonged periods.

Iron

Iron deficiency/insufficiency has been associated with tiredness and fatigue for many decades. Iron is necessary for the manufacture of hemoglobin, the principal oxygen-carrying molecule of red blood cells, and for the activation of many enzyme systems (including energy production). When iron is low, the red cells cannot carry sufficient oxygen to the tissues and we become tired and fatigued. The old sayings "iron-poor blood" and "tired blood" were based upon this understanding.

Doctors used to give iron routinely to people who were tired, especially if they had low blood hemoglobin. Today we know the matter is not so simple. Many other conditions can contribute to low hemoglobin. Moreover, if a person takes iron needlessly it can impair health, since iron can act as an oxidizing agent. This means it can cause free-radical reactions and damage tissue.

A genetic condition known as hemochromatosis affects a large number of people in the U.S. The problem is not too little iron, but an inability to properly utilize and eliminate iron. These individuals suffer easily from iron toxicity, not deficiency. Giving iron to a person with hemochromatosis can lead to serious problems.

Iron overload can lead to hair loss, gastrointestinal problems, altered endocrine function, bone and joint disease, liver problems, and heart disease. Emerging evidence suggests that excessive iron may be a critical factor that predisposes one to heart disease. Ironically, excess iron can contribute to chronic fatigue—much like insufficient iron, but for different reasons.

Some medication can cause iron deficiency, especially in the elderly. Overuse of aspirin, indomethacin, or other antiinflammatory drugs commonly used for arthritic pain may cause bleeding of the intestinal tract, which leads to iron loss.

Iron deficiency/insufficiency can occur at any age. Those most at risk include children under two, adolescent girls, adolescent athletes, athletes who train heavily, menstruating women, and pregnant women. Women with premenstrual syndrome appear to be especially likely to suffer from iron deficiency. If iron deficiency exists in adult men or post-menopausal women, bleeding disorders such as ulcers or cancer should be ruled out. Antiinflammatory drugs such as ibuprofen, which can cause GI bleeding, should also be considered possible culprits.

It may sound confusing, but just remember iron deficiency or iron excess can lead to symptoms of fatigue. Before you or your doctor begin a course of iron supplementation, have your blood checked. A hemoglobin test is not enough. Your doctor should also do a serum ferritin. If the results are still inconclusive, he or she should run an iron profile that includes a few of the tests mentioned below.

Signs and Symptoms

Fatigue	Pale skin, gums, conjunctiva
Brittle nails	Constipation
Irritability	Dizziness
Headaches	Inflamed tongue

Laboratory Tests

Serum ferritin is perhaps the best single test for iron status. Hemoglobin, hematocrit and other blood indices are not tests for iron deficiency. However, if they are altered from the norm, they may cause one to suspect iron deficiency. In some cases, an entire profile is needed to give a clear picture.

- Serum ferritin
- Transferrin saturation (%)
- Total iron binding capacity (TIBC)
- Serum iron

Supplementation

Supplementation with iron is needed when iron deficiency exists. Ferrous gluconate, ferrous peptonate, and ferrous sulfate are commonly used. Many doctors prefer to use forms other than ferrous sulfate. Vitamin C, B_6, folic acid, zinc, and other nutrients enhance iron uptake and utilization.

If your doctor suspects iron deficiency and you have been on an iron supplement without improvement, it is likely that:

1. your problem was not iron deficiency.
2. you have a concurrent nutritional problem or illness.
3. you have an absorption problem that impairs iron uptake into the body, or
4. you are consuming a food, such as coffee, that interferes with iron absorption.

If iron excess or hemochromatosis exist, one method used to reduce levels is frequent donations of blood. This gradually lowers the iron stores in the body. This is called a therapeutic draw and is only done under a doctor's order after the appropriate laboratory tests have been conducted. The drug deferoxamine is sometimes used to lower iron, but some doctors consider the side effects unacceptable.

If you retain anything from this discussion, it should be that both iron deficiency and iron excess can cause chronic fatigue as well as other severe symptoms. You must have your iron status assessed by laboratory methods before embarking on any kind of strategy to alter iron status. Don't just take iron thinking it may be the cause of your fatigue.

Magnesium

Magnesium is needed for many enzyme reactions in the human body. It is vitally important in the production of ATP, the major energy-producing molecule in the body. When magnesium levels are insufficient, energy production suffers and the result can be fatigue. Oddly, magnesium is needed for ATP production, but ATP is needed to get magnesium into the cells. A vicious cycle often develops in fatigued people of low magnesium followed by low ATP (energy) production, which further aggravates magnesium deficiency. It is important to note that the brain has the highest magnesium content, and that many of the symptoms of fatigue are manifested as behavioral or psychological.

In a study of patients with chronic fatigue syndrome, twenty had lower red cell magnesium than did twenty healthy subjects.[20] Dr. D. Dowson, one of the researchers who conducted this study, commented that magnesium therapy was a safe and effective treatment in improving the energy of patients with fatigue. He further commented, "I wouldn't hesitate in using it even if I couldn't check magnesium levels beforehand. We have found it effective in 80 percent of individuals."[21]

William G. Crook, M.D., author of *Chronic Fatigue Syndrome and the Yeast Connection,* conducted an interview in 1991 with Dr. Stephen Davies, editor of the *Journal of Nutritional Medicine.* Davies remarked, "CFS patients are nearly always deficient in magnesium."[22] One of the world's premier researchers of magnesium, Mildred Seelig, reported a study in which magnesium supplementation relieved tiredness in 198 of 200 patients.[23] Sherry Rogers, M.D., showed that after magnesium supplementation, 51 percent of her fatigued patients experienced relief in more than 40 symptoms.[24]

We know magnesium is an important nutrient and that supplementation can improve symptoms of fatigue and tiredness. But how common is magnesium deficiency and what is the dietary intake of the average American? In a survey of more than 27,000 Americans, only 25 percent had a dietary intake of magnesium that equaled or exceeded the RDA.[25] The dietary intake of magnesium for pregnant women in the U.S. is only 35 to 58 percent of the recommended dietary allowance.[26] In one study of people with chemical sensitivity (who also commonly suffer from fatigue), 40 percent were magnesium-deficient.[27]

Signs and Symptoms

Fatigue	Insomnia
Irritability	Muscle spasm or cramps
Easily startled	Anxiety
Confusion	Irregular heartbeat
Noise sensitivity	Restlessness
Rapid heartbeat	Personality changes
Hypertension	

Laboratory Tests

The test for magnesium that appears on your "routine" blood test (often called a SMAC) is a serum magnesium value. Serum magnesium is so closely regulated to protect the heart from fibrillation that it is rarely altered unless there is serious disease. Serum magnesium can be normal even though body stores are depleted. This is because only one percent of the body's magnesium is stored in the blood serum (the liquid part of the blood). The rest lies in blood cells, bone, and other cells. Better indicators of magnesium status include:

- Red blood cell magnesium
- Urinary magnesium loading test
- Urine or plasma amino acid analysis

One or more of these three tests should be ordered to best determine magnesium status. If your doctor says he or she checked your magnesium and it's normal, ask if the test was a *serum* magnesium or one of those mentioned above.

Supplementation

Magnesium is usually given by mouth, or intravenously in severe cases or those with multiple chemical sensitivity. Forms given orally include magnesium chloride, magnesium citrate, magnesium gly-cinate, and magnesium taurate. Magnesium sulfate and magnesium chloride can be given by injection. Magnesium oxide and magne-sium hydroxide are sold over the counter, but are more likely to pro-duce diarrhea. All magnesium supplements can produce diarrhea at high levels because magnesium is a smooth muscle relaxer that can relax bowel muscles. Magnesium glycinate is the least likely of all to do this. According to Sidney Baker, M.D., magnesium chlo-ride is a well-utilized form of magnesium, but it is a prescription form of this nutrient.[28]

Dietary sources of magnesium include legumes, nuts, whole grains, soybeans, seaweed, and seafood. Magnesium is the central atom in the chlorophyll molecule, which is the green pigment in plants. Therefore, magnesium is high in dark-green leafy plants (though agricultural chemicals may decrease the amounts measur-ably). In people with chronic fatigue, it is almost impossible to obtain enough magnesium from food. Supplements are usually needed.

Molybdenum

Molybdenum, a trace element needed in small amounts, is crucial to several enzyme processes within cells. It is needed in the detoxi-fication of chemicals called aldehydes. Aldehydes are common chem-ical contaminants found indoors and outdoors. Formaldehyde is one example. Aldehydes are also produced during the detoxication of other chemicals in the body and in the fermentation of dietary sugars by yeast in the intestines.

People who suffer from intestinal candidiasis or candida-related complex often have a problem with the toxic buildup of aldehydes (acetaldehyde) in the blood, which can make them tired, fatigued, confused, and sluggish. These individuals often benefit from molybdenum supplementation because molybdenum activates the aldehyde oxidase enzyme and allows the person to detoxify these compounds.[29]

Likewise, some people exposed to aldehydes such as formaldehyde at home or work, are unable to detoxify for the same reason noted above. Molybdenum supplementation can be helpful in these cases as well. In multiple chemical sensitivity, molybdenum is often low, which leads to poor tolerance of environmental chemicals. People who are sensitive to sulfites in food (a common additive) can often be helped by molybdenum (plus B_{12} and folic acid).

Signs and Symptoms

Signs and symptoms of molybdenum insufficiency are not clearly established. Symptoms that might cause one to be suspicious of molybdenum insufficiency might include:[30]

Diverse allergy-like symptoms   Sulfite intolerance
Formaldehyde intolerance   Multiple chemical sensitivity
Caffeine intolerance

Laboratory Tests

- Hair molybdenum
- Urine sulfite
- Serum uric acid (if low)

Supplementation

Molybdenum is given when tests suggest it is deficient. Therapeutic amounts are often between 200 and 700 micrograms. Molybdenum should not be taken by someone with gout. Molybdenum content of food can vary by up to 500 percent depending on soil conditions. Foods containing molybdenum include meats, whole grains, leafy vegetables, organ meats, and legumes.

Pantothenic Acid

Pantothenic acid is normally abundant in the body and is involved in numerous biochemical functions. It is part of a compound known as coenzyme A, which is the first molecule in the citric acid cycle— the major energy pathway in the body. Pantothenic acid is also necessary for formation of cortisol in the adrenal glands. Poor adrenal function is a well-known cause of fatigue. When pantothenic acid is given (along with vitamin B_6), adrenal function and energy often improve.

In a study of healthy men, one group received a diet containing pantothenic acid, while the other received a diet without pantothenic acid. Those on the low pantothenate diet became listless and fatigued after only ten weeks.[31]

Pantothenic acid is widely distributed in food. However, food processing has reduced the pantothenic acid content of some people's diets. In general, pantothenic acid insufficiency rarely occurs alone, but insufficiency may occur in combination with other nutrient deficiencies.

Laboratory Tests

- Whole blood pantothenic acid. This test is not commonly ordered. Doctors often give pantothenic acid and observe for improvement in symptoms.

Supplementation

Pantothenic acid is usually given in therapeutic doses between 50 and 800 mg. Daily dietary intake should be around 5 to 7 mg. Forms often used include calcium pantothenate and pantothenic acid, though pantothenic acid is not very stable.

The word "pantos" means "everywhere" and reflects the wide distribution of pantothenic acid in the food supply. It is found in meat, chicken, eggs, fish, cheese, whole grains, nuts, beans, and greens. Fruits and processed foods are not good sources.

Vitamin B_1 (Thiamin)

Dr. Derrick Lonsdale is one of the leading authorities on the role of thiamin in health and disease, and on its role in metabolism. In one study, he found mild vitamin B_1 deficiency in many teenagers who complained of fatigue and irritability. When they were supplemented with B_1, most experienced improvement in energy.[32] When people with fibromyalgia, a painful muscle condition associated with chronic fatigue, were given a form of B_1 (thiamin pyrophosphate), their muscle pain improved significantly.[33]

Thiamin is very important in the body's production of energy. It is necessary in the conversion of blood sugar into energy. If thiamin is low, certain sugars can accumulate in the blood at levels far above normal. Thiamin is also necessary for the body's removal of toxic substances by virtue of its effect on formation of a substance called NADP, which helps to regenerate the important antioxidant glutathione. Without adequate thiamin, the energy and detoxication pathways of the body do not work efficiently.

Signs and Symptoms

Fatigue	Irritability
Memory loss	Nervousness
Weakness	Shortness of breath
Digestive disturbance	Constipation
Depression	Numbness of hands and feet
Pain sensitivity	Confusion

Severe thiamin deficiency can cause massive personality changes, fatigue, and skin problems.

Laboratory Tests

Tests for thiamin status include:[34]

- Erythrocyte transketolase (ETK)
- Thiamin pyrophosphate

Supplementation

Vitamin B_1 is usually given as thiamin HCl (thiamin hydrochloride), thiamin mononitrate, or thiamin pyrophosphate. A therapeutic dosage is around 10 to 100 mg per day. Doctors may give more if they have established a need. Thiamin is found in high concentrations in pork (though I have difficulty recommending pork as a food source). Other sources include nuts, whole grains, legumes, and beans. Dairy products, enriched flour products, and processed foods are poor sources.

Vitamin B_6 (Pyridoxine)

Pyridoxine, or vitamin B_6, is essential for the metabolism of all amino acids. The manufacture of various brain chemicals such as serotonin and dopamine is dependent upon B_6. Vitamin B_6 is also important in protecting against chemical overload and in detoxifying foreign chemicals. It is necessary for active REM sleep, or the period during which we dream. This may be why B_6-deficient people often have trouble remembering dreams and why some have difficulty sleeping. In all, vitamin B_6 is necessary for the function of more than sixty different enzyme reactions in the body. This may be why B_6 needs are so high and why deficiency affects so many body systems. One important symptom of B_6 deficiency is fatigue and low energy. Another is insomnia, which can lead secondarily to fatigue.

In a government study of almost 12,000 adults aged 19 to 74, 90 percent of women and 71 percent of men consumed less than the RDA for vitamin B_6.[35] Selected groups of people are especially likely to suffer from B_6 deficiency. Dr. William Rea reports that 60 percent of chemically sensitive patients are B_6-deficient (based on blood tests), whether or not they are taking B_6 supplements.[36] Thirty-two percent of elderly Americans were also found to have low blood levels of B_6.[37] B_6 was found to be marginally deficient in 50 percent of pregnant women, and it was estimated that a supplement of 20 mg per day may be needed to keep the blood levels of B_6 normal.[38]

Signs and Symptoms

The signs and symptoms of B_6 deficiency are quite general. The main indications include:

Fatigue	Weakness
Mental confusion	Irritability
Nervousness	Insomnia
Skin lesions	Hyperactivity
Anemia	Depression
Tongue and mouth sores	Numbness

Laboratory Tests

- EGOT (erythrocyte glutamate-oxaloacetate transaminase)
- Pyridoxal-5-phosphate (plasma)
- Amino acid analysis of blood or urine

Supplementation

Vitamin B_6 is widely available in over-the-counter form. Pyridoxal-5-phosphate is a form often used by health professionals. Pyridoxine hydrochloride is a common form available in health food stores. In studies where high levels of B_6 were given (>2,000 mg/day), neurological symptoms developed in some patients. This is believed to occur because B_6 was given alone without riboflavin and other B-vitamins. Moreover, two thousand milligrams is an excessive dosage for anyone. Ten to 200 milligrams is considered a therapeutic dose. Nursing mothers who take more than 150 to 200 mg may suppress lactation and decrease their milk supply. People on L-dopa should not take B_6 unless prescribed by a doctor, since B_6 can suppress the action of this drug given for Parkinson's disease.

Food sources of B_6 include meat, poultry, egg yolk, fish, peanuts, walnuts, and dried beans. Whole grain cereals, bananas, potatoes, cabbage, avocados, and cauliflower are other good sources.

Vitamin B$_{12}$ (Cobalamin)

B$_{12}$ deficiency is a well-known cause of fatigue. Dr. H. L. Newbold has reported on his use of B$_{12}$ in the treatment of fatigue for more than 20 years. He notes improvement even in patients with normal serum B$_{12}$ levels. Physician and researcher Stephen Davies has commented on a study entitled "Neuropsychiatric disorders caused by cobalamin (Vitamin B$_{12}$) deficiency in the absence of anemia or macrocytosis."[39,40] Davies states:

"It is interesting that fatigue was common in the absence of anemia but this cleared on cobalamin [vitamin B$_{12}$] therapy; this observation is reminiscent of the report by Ellis et al[41] who conducted a double blind trial of cobalamin administration showing it [B$_{12}$] to be more effective than placebo in the treatment of 'tiredness' for which no other physical cause could be found. In Ellis' study, no subject was included in the trial whose initial serum B$_{12}$ values were not in the normal range."

Alexander Bralley, Ph.D., whose laboratory is engaged in several studies of patients with chronic fatigue, reported to me in 1993 that roughly 50 percent of their tests of fatigued patients show elevated methylmalonic acid, meaning vitamin B$_{12}$ deficiency.[42]

Conventional wisdom holds that vitamin B$_{12}$ is stored for prolonged periods in the body and that it takes many years to develop deficiency. However, B$_{12}$ deficiency may be more common than previously thought, in part because of marked decline of B$_{12}$ in foodstuffs. Dr. Russell Jaffe has reviewed a series of factors that have given rise to this dramatic decrease in the availability of B$_{12}$ in the diet. He notes, for instance, that in the 1960s, beef liver contained 122 micrograms (mcg) of B$_{12}$ per 100 grams (g). Tests done in 1990 detected no B$_{12}$ in beef liver. In the 1960s, beef heart contained 14 mcg per 100 g. Tests done in 1990 found only 2 mcg per 100 g. In the 1960s, Swiss cheese was reported to contain 0.5 mcg of B$_{12}$ per 100 g. In 1990, none was detected. Egg yolk dropped from 9 mcg in the 1960s to 1 mcg in 1990.[43]

These dramatic declines in B$_{12}$ do not bode well for our present and future health. Much of the decline has been attributed to the use of chemicals in agriculture, and to the overuse of antibiotics in medicine and animal husbandry.

Why do antibiotics affect vitamin B_{12} production? Primarily because this vitamin is a product of bacterial fermentation. Bacteria in the digestive tracts of cattle and humans are a primary source. Cheese, cultured dairy products, and fermented foods such as miso also contribute some B_{12}. Since antibiotics destroy bacteria or cause them to alter their metabolism, many researchers believe that antibiotic overuse has in part contributed to the decline in B_{12}.

Anyone can develop B_{12} insufficiency or deficiency. Strict vegetarians and those on a macrobiotic diet are perhaps most at risk. Those with intestinal illness, parasites, malabsorption and other diseases of the ileum or colon are also at risk. Those with irritable bowel syndrome are commonly B_{12} deficient as are the elderly. Due to the general decline of B_{12} in the food chain, B_{12} insufficiency may occur in other groups.

Signs and symptoms

Weakness	Fatigue
Dizziness	Irritability
Sore tongue	Depression
Memory impairment	Moodiness
Confusion	Paleness

Laboratory Tests

Serum B_{12} tests commonly used today are not as sensitive as the newer tests such as methylmalonic acid.

- Methylmalonic acid (24-hour urine)
- Urinary or plasma homocystine (barring B_6 and folate deficiency)
- Neutrophil hypersegmentation index

Supplementation

Vitamin B_{12} is usually given by injection in the United States. In countries such as Sweden, about 40 percent of those needing B_{12} are given oral supplements. Oral supplements are satisfactory for many cases of B_{12} deficiency.[44] Vitamin B_{12} status should be monitored by a doctor. If there are neurological symptoms such as numbness, tingling, or loss of vibratory sensation, a doctor's advice is especially important.

Vitamin C

Vitamin C is important in immune function, manufacture of connective tissue (the stuff that holds us together), detoxication of drugs and chemicals, protection against foreign chemicals, and many other functions. Deficiency of vitamin C has also been associated with fatigue. Since about 1750, it has been known that many sailors on long voyages became fatigued and eventually died. It was later discovered that this was due to vitamin C deficiency, which led to a condition called scurvy. Fatigue seems to develop within about 90 days of beginning a diet low in vitamin C.

Physician and researcher Emmanuel Cheraskin, M.D., D.M.D., conducted a study several years ago that evaluated the vitamin C intakes of 411 dentists and their spouses. Cheraskin looked at the number of fatigue symptoms each person listed when taking the Cornell Medical Index Health Questionnaire and compared them with daily vitamin C intake. It was discovered that those consuming less than 100 mg of vitamin C per day had a fatigability score twice that of those consuming 400 mg or more of vitamin C per day.[45] In other words, those with the highest intakes of vitamin C reported fewer fatigue symptoms.

The benefits of vitamin C in protection against cancer, heart disease, infections, and other conditions continue to be published in the medical literature.

Signs and Symptoms

Fatigue	Bleeding gums
Easy bruising	Tiredness
Malaise	Loose teeth
Poor wound healing	Depression
Infections	Frequent colds

Laboratory Tests

Since there is such a wide safety range for vitamin C, doctors often prescribe this nutrient without running blood tests. There is no single ideal test of vitamin C that is suitable in all situations. Tests currently used include:[46]

- Plasma vitamin C
- Leukocyte (white blood cell) vitamin C: reflects vitamin C status over a slightly longer period time than plasma.
- Urine ascorbate.
- Lingual ascorbic acid test—a useful, inexpensive screening test.

Supplementation

Vitamin C has a wide margin of safety. The main questions are how much does one take and in what form. Dosage depends upon severity of symptoms. Common forms include mineral ascorbates where the ascorbic acid is buffered with trace minerals—usually calcium, zinc, magnesium, sodium, and potassium. This form is less likely to cause diarrhea than ascorbic acid. Buffered forms of vitamin C can also be taken at higher doses without concern of leaching trace elements from the body. Ester-C, which was developed in the 1980s, has been shown to be taken up more rapidly into white blood cells, and therefore may be a very good oral source of vitamin C.

Zinc

Zinc is essential for immune function, regulating inflammation, protecting against toxic exposure, detoxifying foreign chemicals, digestive function, and numerous other body functions. It is also essential for taste and smell. Zinc is required for activity of the enzyme lactic dehydrogenase. This enzyme is needed to eliminate lactic acid from muscles after they are used for physical activity. If zinc levels are insufficient, lactic acid builds up more easily, muscles are easily fatigued, and muscle pain is more common.

Zinc is also a cofactor in the enzyme alcohol dehydrogenase, which helps in detoxifying alcohol and certain chemical toxins with alcohol groups. Dr. Sherry Rogers describes a case of a woman with persistent headaches and chronic fatigue that lasted for 11 years despite all forms of medical intervention. Dr. Rogers discovered the woman had high blood levels of a chemical called trichloroethylene, which is normally detoxified by the zinc-dependent alcohol dehydrogenase enzyme. Unfortunately, the woman was also zinc-deficient so the enzyme worked inefficiently. After one month of zinc supplementation, her headaches cleared.[47]

Zinc deficiency has been found in some patients who suffer from fatigue. Dr. Stephen Davies has commented that many patients with chronic fatigue syndrome are deficient in zinc. Dr. Carol Jessop, who has treated more than 1,000 patients with chronic fatigue syndrome, notes that 32 percent of her patients with CFS show deficiency of zinc based on blood tests. She also notes that the various blood tests used to assess zinc status are not as accurate as other more difficult tests for zinc status, so the percentage of zinc deficient patients may be much higher than she reports.[48]

Many Americans get inadequate amounts of zinc in their diets. In one study of American men and women, 68 percent were found to consume less than two-thirds of the RDA for zinc.[49] Zinc is also commonly low in the elderly. In one study, zinc intake was below the RDA in more than 90 percent of those aged 60 to 89.[50] The elderly also consume prescription drugs that deplete zinc such as diuretics and cardiac glycosides.

Signs and Symptoms

Fatigue	Irritability
Infections	Depression
Diarrhea	Eczema
Decreased taste	Decreased sense of smell
Poor wound healing	White spots on nails
Lethargy	Memory impairment
Brittle nails	Impotence

Laboratory Tests

Assessment of zinc status is not as clear-cut as for some other nutrients. The best tests include:

- Red cell zinc
- Hair mineral analysis (inverse relationship)
- Perspiration zinc (though not commonly done)
- Lactic dehydrogenase

Supplementation

Zinc supplements come in several different forms. Zinc sulfate, zinc picolinate, and zinc gluconate are commonly used forms of zinc. Common therapeutic dosages range from 25 to 50 mg per day. When zinc is used in high doses or for extended periods it is often given with copper. Zinc can produce decreases in immune function and alteration in blood fats when consumed in excess for several months or years because of competition with copper and iron. Never exceed 50 mg per day for extended periods without the supervision of a health professional knowledgeable in nutrition.

Fruits and vegetables are poor sources of zinc. Animal foods including egg yolk and meat are good sources. Whole grains contain zinc, but zinc is not easily absorbed from whole grains.

Alpha-Lipoic Acid

Alpha-lipoic acid (thioctic acid) is one of the body's most powerful antioxidants. It is unique among antioxidants in that it is both fat-soluble and water-soluble. It has the capability to exert its antioxidant affects in two vastly different domains within the body. Moreover, it has the capability to regenerate other important antioxidants such as vitamin C, vitamin E, coenzyme Q10 and glutathione. In fact, giving lipoic acid actually raises the body's levels of glutathione better than almost any other substance, including glutathione itself. It quenches some of the most dangerous free radicals in the body and prevents peroxidation (damage) of the body's delicate fatty acids.

Lipoic acid is being viewed as one the most promising nutrients for treatment of brain disorders. In fact, it is one nutrient that successfully protects nerve cells from molecules known as excitotoxins. Lipoic acid is vital to the energy pathways in the body's mitochondria. It is important in helping to regulate blood sugar and is involved in fat metabolism. Alpha lipoic acid is being used supplementall for a variety of conditions ranging from diabetic neuropathy to chronic fatigue. In the U.S. it is most widely used for treating diabetes, but in Europe it has been used to treat liver disease and neurological disorders for some time.

Signs and Symptoms

No classic deficiency signs have yet been associated with alpha-lipoic acid

Laboratory Tests

• Lipoic acid

Supplementation

Lipoic acid is given as either lipoic acid or dihydrolipoic acid. Thioctic acid is another name that you may see, but it is not as commonly used. Doses of lipoic acid range from 100 to 600 mg daily. Lipoic acid is among the most expensive of the nutrients. However, it functions in ways that very few antioxidants function. Its influence on the body's energy system is so unique and its ability to increase levels of the vital glutathione molecule so significant that lipoic acid is among the truly prized nutrients for supplementation.

Foods vs. Nutritional Supplements

There is a fundamental debate between doctors with differing nutritional philosophies regarding whether one should attempt to correct nutrient insufficiency by supplementation or through food. It would take some time to discuss all pertinent aspects of this debate, but I would like to leave you with the essence of my opinion.

Food has advantages because it contains many biologically active phytochemicals not encountered in most supplements. A disadvantage of food is that the nutrient levels vary widely depending upon season, storage, preparation, region of growth, and chemical use. Organic food appears to have higher levels of many nutrients than similar commercially grown food. Another disadvantage of food as a primary therapeutic tool is that it may not contain the desired nutrients in sufficient amounts for therapeutic benefit. One may have to consume unobtainable amounts of a food to receive a given amount of a particular nutrient. If one has food intolerance or food allergies, a restrictive diet may be in order that would necessitate supplementation for a period of time. Should intestinal malabsorption exist, far higher levels of nutrients may have to be taken than would normally be necessary or available through food.

In essence, I believe food has enormous therapeutic potential. Specialized therapeutic food regimens have been a staple of ancient healing practices and will remain so for centuries to come. Likewise, supplementation has a critical role to play in both prevention of illness and treatment of illness. I firmly believe that the best therapeutic programs make use of carefully planned therapeutic diets combined with supplementation tailored to the individual's biochemistry. This combination offers the most powerful tool in any health recovery program.

A final note is in order. I believe nutritional supplements *are never a substitute for a well-balanced diet.* They can and should be used to augment a good diet. Food is where the healing begins.

In Conclusion

In this section I have reviewed the principal nutrients that contribute to fatigue and poor energy. In a given case, other nutrients not mentioned here may be involved as well. You may have noticed that there is a great deal of overlap with regard to signs and symptoms. This is because the interaction between nutrients is very complex and there is much interdependence. Recognize also that in many people with chronic fatigue, more than one nutrient deficiency is common. In fact, multiple nutrient deficiencies may be the rule rather than the exception.

This chapter has likely both clarified and confused with regard to the role of nutrients in fatigue. I suggest that you look carefully at the symptoms to determine whether any match your own. You may next wish to work with health a professional who will do the appropriate workup to determine nutritional intake and then actual nutrient levels. Nutrition intake can be assessed using food frequency questionnaires analyzed by computer. Nutrient levels and functional need may be assessed by the laboratory tests discussed above.

Chapter 5

Blood Sugar Disorders

CHRONIC FATIGUE IS a common feature of people with blood sugar problems because sugar is the fuel that runs the brain, the muscles, and other body cells. Without adequate blood sugar regulation, function of many body systems goes awry and poor energy balance is the result. Notice I said poor blood sugar *regulation*. There is hardly any person in this culture who does not eat adequate amounts of sugar. The problem lies in how the body regulates all sugars that enter it.

The two most common forms of blood sugar disorders are hypoglycemia and diabetes. Hypoglycemia occurs when blood sugar levels (which usually refers to the sugar glucose) rise and fall at irregular rates and affect metabolism of energy. It generally means low blood glucose. With low blood glucose comes low energy, sleepiness, tiredness, difficulty concentrating, poor memory, and irritability. Diabetes is a problem of insulin production or utilization. Insulin is a hormone produced by the pancreas that regulates the amount of glucose circulating in the blood. Diabetics have a problem with elevated blood glucose. When blood glucose is too high, a very dangerous situation exists in which the body's metabolism can be severely disrupted.

Both blood sugar disorders can cause fatigue and are closely tied to trace mineral status and diet.[1] Overconsumption of sugar is an important dietary cause of blood sugar abnormalities in this culture. Soda pop serves as an excellent example to illustrate this point. The resting blood glucose of an eight-year-old boy is about 100 (mg/dl), which means that at any given time he has about one teaspoon of glucose circulating in his blood. The average can of carbonated cola contains eight to nine teaspoons of sugar. If this boy drinks a can of pop, his blood is hit with a dose of sugar that is *eight or nine times* its normal resting levels. In response, the body must mobilize large amounts of adrenalin and insulin to clear the sugar from the bloodstream. Repeated day after day, this scenario can lead to significant health problems, not the least of which is blood sugar disorders.

To put this in perspective, consider the following discoveries about the yearly consumption habits of the average American with regard to sugar:[2]

- 134 pounds of refined sugar excluding honey
- 365 servings of soda pop (638 cans per year for people aged 12–29)
- 200 sticks of gum
- 22 pounds of candy
- 63 dozen doughnuts
- 60 pounds of cakes and cookies
- 23 gallons of ice cream

Let's take our soda pop analogy a step further. Colas are strongly acidic. To solve this problem, manufacturers add phosphoric acid as a buffer. Unfortunately, phosphoric acid binds to magnesium. Consumption of one can of cola containing phosphoric acid can cause a subsequent loss of 36 milligrams of magnesium from the body. Recall the studies mentioned earlier pointing out the importance of magnesium deficiency in chronic fatigue. Magnesium is vitally important in energy metabolism. If this magnesium is not replaced, the gradual depletion can lead to a variety of health problems.

Diabetes is separated into two major types. In type I, which usually affects children and young adults, the insulin-producing cells in the pancreas are destroyed. Insulin is necessary to regulate blood glucose so these people—about 500,000 in the United States—must receive daily doses of insulin. Failure to properly regulate insulin and blood glucose levels can lead to serious consequences.

There is evidence that some cases of type I diabetes may be triggered by early introduction of cow's milk into an infant's diet.[3] This suggests that some cases of diabetes may be due to an autoimmune reaction in which the immune system attacks the pancreatic cells that produce insulin.

In type II diabetes, often called adult-onset diabetes, the body usually makes either too much or too little insulin. Moreover, there is a problem with insulin responsiveness of the body cells. Type II diabetes affects an estimated 12 million people in the United States. These individuals are often treated with diet, oral hypoglycemic drugs, or insulin. Many sufferers of type II diabetes do not require insulin. Exercise and weight loss are very important and very helpful. Good nutrition is essential.

Many doctors do not give adequate attention given to the status of the trace element chromium in people with blood sugar disorders. Studies as far back as the 1960s showed chromium deficiency to be associated with poor insulin regulation and diabetes. In 1968, Dr. K. Hambridge showed that diabetic children had significantly lower chromium levels than normal children.[4] An article that appeared in the *Southern Medical Journal* in 1977 entitled "Chromium Depletion in the Pathogenesis of Diabetes and Atherosclerosis" showed that deficiency of chromium was a prime factor in the cause of these disorders.[5] One reason sugar may trigger blood sugar problems is it may actually increase the amount of chromium that is spilled into the urine and therefore lost.[6]

Other nutrients are being investigated in diabetes. A study published in *Clinical Chemistry* showed children with insulin-dependent diabetes had lower levels of magnesium than normal children.[7] In another study, non-insulin-dependent diabetic adults with microangiopathy (a blood vessel complication) had elevated blood homocysteine, which is one indicator of possible vitamin B_{12} deficiency.

Injections of B_{12} (methylcobalamin) improved their blood homocysteine levels.[8]

Vitamin C has also been studied with regard to its role in blood
sugar disorders. The molecular structures of glucose (a sugar) and
ascorbic acid (vitamin C) are very similar. Some scientists believe
that sugar and vitamin C compete for uptake into cells, and that
excess sugar in the diet may disrupt the normal transport of vitamin C into cells. This might result in altered repair functions, decreased immunity, and altered inflammatory response.[9] Vitamin C
has been found to enhance insulin action and may reduce some of
the blood vessel complications of diabetes.[10]

Alan Gaby and Jonathan Wright reviewed the nutrients involved
in blood sugar disorders in their paper "Nutritional Regulation of
Blood Glucose," published in the *Journal of Advancement in Medicine* in 1991. Nutrients discussed include chromium, niacin, biotin,
pyridoxine, copper, magnesium, potassium, zinc, manganese, vitamin C, selenium, vitamin B_{12}, folic acid, thiamin, calcium, carnitine, vanadium, and vitamin E.[11] Alpha-lipoic acid has been found
to have a significant impact on improving blood sugar metabolism.
In addition, it is a powerful antioxidant that can even benefit neuropathy when blood sugar disorders such as diabetes have advanced.

Food intolerance also plays a role in the blood sugar problems of
some people. In the *Basics of Food Allergy* by James C. Breneman,
M.D., food sensitivities were reported to cause 75 percent of all functional hypoglycemia.[12] One of my former patients illustrates this point.
An 11-year-old boy had diabetes for which he was receiving insulin.
The problem was that his doctors could not seem to stabilize his blood
glucose no matter how they manipulated his insulin. I identified a
sensitivity to corn as a possible contributor. His blood glucose rose
far beyond normal levels after a dose of corn. After eliminating corn
from his diet, his blood glucose was more easily regulated. He still
required some insulin, but only a fraction of what was once needed.

It is not possible to do justice to the subject of blood sugar disorders in a book as brief as this. Recognize, however, that blood sugar
problems do contribute to fatigue. A few simple tests can rule this
in or out in your case.

Signs and Symptoms of Hypoglycemia

Fatigue	Tiredness
Mood swings	Nervousness
Dizziness	Rapid heart beat (some)

Symptoms typically begin three to five hours after a meal. If they begin within zero to three hours of a meal, consider food allergy or a high tryptophan/high carbohydrate diet as the cause.

Signs and Symptoms of Diabetes

Below are some of the warning signs that type I diabetes may exist.

Fatigue	Frequent urination
Excessive thirst	Recurrent blurred vision
Numbness	Vaginal itching in women
Weight loss	

Type II diabetes is commonly associated with the following symptoms:

Fatigue
Excessive weight or weight gain
Recurrent infections of skin and urinary tract
Itching of skin and genitals

In chronic diabetes the signs are more serious and more evident. They include some of the following:

Changes in sensation of the extremities
Changes in the blood vessels of the arms and legs
Chronic skin lesions
Visual changes such as cataracts

Laboratory Tests

- Urine glucose
- Blood glucose

- Glucose tolerance test (There is disagreement over the value of this test.)
- Insulin tolerance test
- Glycosylated hemoglobin (HbA1c)
- AGE (advanced glycation endproducts)
- Red blood cell chromium
- Hair chromium level
- Other trace elements and vitamins as indicated

If you have a blood sugar disorder and have not had your nutrient status checked, you have not done your detective work. Ask your doctor (or find one who will work with you) to check your red blood cell and hair chromium in addition to other nutrients.

Treatment

Treatment of blood sugar disorders is highly individual, but does involve some basic similarities. Diabetes is usually treated with insulin, oral hypoglycemic drugs, and dietary management. Exercise and therapeutic nutrition are also being used by some doctors. Chromium is especially important.

The antihypoglycemia diet places emphasis on five areas:

1. High fiber
2. High protein
3. Low carbohydrate
4. Avoidance of refined sugars
5. Avoidance of food allergens

The general diet used in diabetes emphasizes:

1. High fiber
2. Balance between protein:fat:carbohydrate of roughly 40 percent, 30 percent, 30 percent
3. Restriction of refined sugar
4. Avoidance of food allergens

The American Diabetes Association has begun to alter their guidelines for diabetics based on whether the individual has type I or type II, whether they are obese or overweight, or whether they have elevated blood fats. Other changes have been made as well. It has become clear that sugar alone acts differently than sugar and fat combined, and that the type of sugar is extremely important. For example, glucose and fructose have very different effects on blood sugar. Pure glucose has a glycemic index of 100, whereas fructose is only 20. Moreover, a food such as potato has a less dramatic effect on blood sugar when consumed with fat of some form, since fat can slow the rate at which glucose is delivered to the blood. The new guidelines allow for a less restrictive diet with regard to sugars as long as the diet is appropriately balanced and tailored to the individual needs. More recent opinion of diabetes suggests that the balance between protein, fat, and carbohydrate is very important and argues for a roughly 40:30:30 balance.

Exercise can be of great benefit in blood sugar disorders. This is especially true of hypoglycemia and non-insulin-dependent diabetes mellitus. A 1992 review of several scientific papers on diabetes and exercise showed a clear benefit in regulating blood sugar.[13] Those with insulin-dependent diabetes (IDDM) did not show improved blood sugar regulation following exercise. However, exercise is still important in IDDM because of the benefits to cardiovascular health and fat metabolism. Exercise in IDDM should only be undertaken with the supervision of a doctor.

In Review

1. Blood sugar disorders can affect mood and energy.
2. Hypoglycemia and diabetes are the two most common blood sugar disorders.
3. Dietary manipulation and nutritional supplementation can be an important part of improving blood sugar regulation.
4. Exercise also helps the body regulate its blood sugar.

Chapter 6

Elevated Blood Fats

TRIGLYCERIDES AND CHOLESTEROL are called blood fats or blood lipids. When these and related blood lipids are too high, it can impair the transport of oxygen through the blood and result in easy fatigability. Moreover, if elevated blood fats are coupled with deficiency of antioxidant nutrients and imbalance of essential fatty acids, damage to blood vessels can occur, which further restricts the flow of oxygen. People with elevated blood lipids are frequently tired, fatigue easily, and are often in poor aerobic condition. When blood lipid levels return to normal, energy often improves (not to mention a lower risk of heart disease and other degenerative diseases).

Jeremy is a good example. He was a 51-year-old businessman who had a cholesterol of 356 and a triglyceride level of 600. He wasn't careful about his diet and didn't exercise at all. On the few occasions his wife was able to coax him out for a walk, he became winded after a 15-minute turn around the block. He was tired all the time and took naps frequently, yet he never seemed to have much energy.

He had been taking medication to lower his blood fats, but this seemed to be having only a marginal effect. I placed him on L-carnitine, chromium, EPA (fish oil), and lipotrophic factors such as methionine, choline, and inositol for several months. Without much change in diet, his blood fats returned to near normal and his fatigue diminished substantially.

Another man, Rick, had blood fats in nearly the same range as Jeremy. When I looked at his blood through a dark-field microscope, the white-colored triglycerides were so high it looked like a snow-storm. In one month of taking L-carnitine, chromium, other lipo-trophic nutrients, and EPA, his lipids returned to normal and his fatigue cleared.

Elevation of blood fats is one of the most common health prob-lems in America and a major contributor to heart disease. Elevated blood fats can also contribute to sluggish immunity. This is because when fat levels get too high, the ability of white blood cells to engulf and destroy bacteria drops dramatically. Jeremy also "caught" every cold and flu bug that seemed to be going around. This all changed when he finally got his blood lipids under control.

An important consideration in the blood fat problem is the level of antioxidant nutrients such as vitamin E, vitamin C, alpha-carotene, beta-carotene, lycopene, coenzyme Q, and vitamin A. All lipids are subject to damage by free radicals that are generated from normal bodily processes or encountered in the environment. Lipids that become damaged by free radicals are more apt to be involved in development of a disease process. A certain amount of antioxidant nutrient reserve is required to protect the lipids in the body from oxidative damage. As the levels of blood lipids go up, the amount of antioxidant nutrients required to protect them from damage increases as well.

For example, one molecule of vitamin E protects roughly 1,000 molecules of cholesterol. If cholesterol levels go up while vitamin E levels go down, the risk to damaged blood fats increases. Moreover, vitamin C is able to regenerate vitamin E indicating a complex inter-action among antioxidants. In general, those with higher blood lipids need more antioxidants to protect them. The problem is, the dietary and lifestyle habits that lead to development of elevated blood fats are often habits that provide *inadequate* amounts of antioxidant nutrients. For these and other reasons, it is helpful to check the blood antioxidant levels as well as blood lipids.

More research is beginning to focus on the problem of trans fatty acids and their effect on blood fats and heart disease. Recall that trans fatty acids result when unsaturated oils have been heated, exposed to oxygen, or processed. Indeed, recent evidence suggests that trans fatty acid consumption (such as from margarine or deep-fried foods) may be a more important contributor to heart disease than saturated fat. According to an article in the *American Journal of Public Health*, "There is strong evidence that trans fatty acids are causally related to coronary disease. The number of deaths attributed to the consumption of trans fats is considerable."[1] This important discovery (which has actually been suspected for decades) will undoubtedly receive much attention in the coming years. Trans fatty acids cause enormous metabolic problems and should be avoided as much as possible.

Laboratory Tests

The following tests are considered part of a thorough assessment of blood fats.

- Total serum cholesterol
- HDL (high density lipoprotein)
- LDL (low density lipoprotein)
- Serum triglycerides
- Apolipoprotein B
- Cholesterol/HDL ratio
- LDL/Apolipoprotein B ratio
- Essential fatty acids analysis (including an analysis for trans fatty acids)

Tests of antioxidant status are important because they reflect the degree to which the body and cell lipids (fats) are protected from free radical damage. Tests for fat-soluble antioxidants include:

- Coenzyme Q_{10} (ubiquinol)
- Alpha-tocopherol (vitamin E)
- Gamma-tocopherol
- Lycopene

- Beta-carotene
- Alpha-carotene
- Vitamin A

Tests for water-soluble antioxidants include:

- Ascorbic acid
- Uric acid
- Bilirubin

The above tests for antioxidants can be enormously helpful in understanding blood fat abnormalities and, equally important, devising a nutrient plan aimed at restoring health. Pantox Laboratories in San Diego currently offers such tests. (See list of laboratories in Appendix.)

Treatment

Nutrients that aid in lowering cholesterol include: methionine, choline, inositol, betaine, B_{12}, folic acid, taurine, B_6, vitamin C, magnesium, and vitamin E.

Nutrients that aid in lowering triglycerides include: Those listed above with the addition of L-carnitine (which is essential for oxidation of free fatty acids), EPA/DHA, and chromium.

The dietary recommendations surrounding elevated blood fats have changed markedly over the past several years. It was once thought that excess dietary cholesterol was a big part of the problem. This view is giving way to a new view that contends it is the oxidized form of cholesterol in the diet coupled with excess saturated fat, excess sugar, and deficient levels of antioxidants that contribute to the blood fat problem.

Trans fatty acids should be avoided at all costs. They serve no purpose in the body and only appear to do harm. Ironically, physicians who recommended margarine over butter many years ago to prevent heart disease may have inadvertently contributed to the problem they attempted to remedy. Why? Margarine is high in trans fatty acids.

In attempting to improve blood fat levels one should always incorporate exercise into dietary and nutritional programs. This is because both aerobic exercise and weight training serve to increase HDL (which you want) and decrease LDL (which you also want to do). Exercise should be initiated carefully and should always be tailored to your individual health and fitness level. You should see your doctor about exercise that is appropriate for your existing level of health.

In Review

1. Elevated blood fats can contribute to fatigue.
2. Elevated blood fats can impair circulation and lower immunity.
3. Antioxidant nutrients are needed to protect lipids from damage by free radicals.
4. Dietary changes and nutritional supplementation can help many people with elevated blood fats.

Chapter 7

Overweight and Underlean: How Those Extra Pounds Can Cause Fatigue

PEOPLE WHO ARE overweight may complain of fatigue for many different reasons. If you are overweight you may be at greater risk to diabetes, high blood pressure, heart disease, and lowered immunity, all associated with chronic fatigue. Being overweight can also restrict the movement of the diaphragm, thus restricting your breathing. When you are unable to take regular, deep, diaphragmatic breaths, you transport less oxygen to the tissues and may suffer from fatigue and sluggishness. Lowered thyroid function, another cause of fatigue, is also somewhat common among overweight people.

Excessive weight may sometimes be due to food allergy or food intolerance. When an individual is consuming foods to which he or she is allergic, immune complexes may form that circulate throughout the bloodstream. One way the body attempts to minimize the impact of such a reaction is to retain fluid. In essence, the body tries to dilute these complexes by making them less concentrated. The excess fluid then contributes to extra girth and weight.

One reason people on weight-loss diets lose weight so quickly is they reduce their intake of allergenic foods. This leads to the loss of water from tissue spaces. This kind of weight loss is only temporary and has little effect on body fat. Identifying foods to which you may be sensitive or allergic should be a part of any weight-reduction program, but additional elements are needed.

Adding to the problem of excessive weight is the fact that most environmental toxins are fat-soluble, meaning they dissolve easily in fat tissue. Because of this, fat acts like a storage house for the chemicals with which you come in contact. This can make dieting to lose weight a tricky matter because when you begin to burn off fat, stored toxins may be released back into the bloodstream. This can cause a barrage of symptoms including headaches, dizziness, muscle aches, fatigue, and many others. Thus, any weight-reduction program should be coupled with intake of nutrients that enhance the body's detoxication mechanism. This reduces the chance that toxic reexposure will cause harm as fat is being lost.

Excess consumption of sugar and simple carbohydrates is a considerable problem for people who are overweight or underlean. Excess sugar in the diet gets converted into fat and is stored in fat cells. This is true for fruit-based sugars as well as table sugar. Consumption of too much fat in the wrong form can contribute to the poor energy metabolism often associated with being overweight and appears to contribute to some of the other associated problems such as hypertension, diabetes, and blood vessel diseases. Those who are overweight often consume too much of the following fats:

- Trans fatty acids: found in french fries, chicken nuggets, and other deep-fried foods; margarine; potato chips; cookies and candies; baked goods such as doughnuts.
- Saturated fat: found in animal products such as beef, pork, and dairy products.
- Omega-6 fatty acids: found in corn oil, sunflower oil, safflower oil, and sesame oil.

Overweight/underlean individuals often consume too little of the following fats:

- Omega-3 fatty acids: found in flax oil, walnut oil, and pumpkin seed oil; in animals such as salmon, mackerel, herring, sardines, and other cold water fish.
- Monounsaturated fatty acids: found in olive oil.

When being overweight is a result of consuming excessive calories, it can lead to a noticeable decrease in immune function. Paul Newbern and Pamela Williams, formerly of the Massachusetts Institute of Technology, have shown that dogs raised on high-calorie diets were more likely to succumb to infection by canine distemper virus and salmonella bacteria. Those with the highest caloric intakes were more likely to suffer from encephalitis as a result of canine distemper virus infection[1] It is fairly well established that excessive caloric intake can lower immunity and impair health. The real paradox is that very often, people who are overweight actually consume fewer calories than those who are lean and fit. Unfit people with high body fat burn calories much less efficiently than fit people with low body fat.

If you are overweight/underlean, you should be put on a well-regulated program that includes:

- Adequate protein, moderate calorie diet
- Metabolic detoxification
- Low allergen diet
- Nutritional support
- Exercise

You should avoid programs that:

- Waste muscle (many do)
- Restrict calories

Some doctors are beginning to use the term *underlean* rather than overweight. This refers to the fact that most people who are above their ideal body weight suffer from a lack of lean muscle mass and an excess of body fat. In essence, their lean body mass to body fat ratio is too low. The goal then is to increase lean muscle mass and decrease body fat.

Jeffrey S. Bland, Ph.D., and his colleagues conducted a study in which they compared a doctor-supervised program aimed at improving lean body mass with a popular, unsupervised, over-the-counter (OTC) weight loss program. Those on the popular OTC program experienced:[2]

- A significant adverse alteration in thyroid function
- An average loss of only one pound of fat (though more than one pound of weight was actually lost)
- Muscle loss

The people on the doctor-supervised program experienced:

- No adverse change in thyroid function
- Loss of an average of 10 pounds of fat
- No loss of muscle

The problem with most people who are overfat is that their metabolism is sluggish. You must attempt to increase your metabolism by changing the foods you eat and by exercising.

One cannot overemphasize the importance of exercise in losing weight, improving lean muscle mass, losing fat, and improving energy. One study looked at the effect of exercise without dietary restrictions on overweight people. In six month's time, those who walked or rode a stationary bicycle (60 minutes per day) lost 10 percent and 12 percent respectively of their initial body weight. For a 150-pound person that translates into roughly a 15-pound weight loss *without* going on a diet; for a 200-pound person, a loss of 20 pounds.[3]

When dietary restriction was compared to exercise as a means to reduce weight, researchers discovered that dietary restriction alone actually *decreased* the resting metabolic rate and decreased lean muscle mass. A decrease in resting metabolic rate is significant since this accounts for 70 to 75 percent of daily energy expenditure.[4] In essence, calorie restriction alone appears to lessen the efficiency with which the body burns fuel for energy.

Princeton University researchers conclude that exercise is critical to weight loss because it:[5]

- May help to increase resting metabolic rate
- Increases activation of the sympathetic nervous system
- Increases activation of brown fat (which is desirable)

- Increases release of growth hormone (necessary for building muscle)
- Ensures that fat weight is lost and not muscle
- May lead to lingering calorie expenditure after the exercise is stopped
- Can improve insulin resistance

Not all people who are overweight or underlean suffer from poor energy. However, anyone who is overweight can improve the efficiency of their metabolism by combining exercise with proper nutrition and food consumption.

Laboratory Tests

Since being overweight and underlean is often associated with metabolic imbalance and poor nutrient status, tests to assess these parameters should be considered. Your doctor should also do an examination to rule out any medical conditions such as pituitary, thyroid, or cardiovascular problems that might be responsible for the excessive weight/fat or that might necessitate a reduced or modified exercise program.

You should also have a body fat analysis performed. This will give you an indication of your lean body mass. Once you know your percent body fat, you can begin a program geared toward lowering it.

Ideal Percentage Body Fat for Men and Women

Men	14–18%
Women	19–23%

Body fat is usually measured using underwater immersion testing, skin fold thickness, electrical impedance, or infrared measurement of a muscle group. Each test has its pros and cons. The skin fold thickness is commonly done and is inexpensive. The infrared measurement is easily done, reproducible, and gives a reasonable assessment. Underwater immersion requires sophisticated equipment that most facilities do not have.

Remember, while weight may be your immediate concern, you should be most concerned about body fat. Don't worry about the scale and how many pounds you have shed. Focus instead on your beginning body fat percentage and upon reducing that number.

You should be aware that many people who go on a *fat*-reduction program that is coupled with exercise (unless they are extremely overweight) may actually *gain* weight or stay the same. Don't be discouraged by this. When fat is lost and replaced by muscle, you may actually weigh more because muscle is heavier than fat. It is not the overall weight that is critical, but the percent body fat. This one reason measuring body fat is so important.

Treatment

The treatment for the overweight/overfat/underlean individual involves two important aspects: controlled *fat*-reduction program and exercise. If you do one without the other, you won't experience the level of success you might desire. If you embark on a weight-reduction or fat-reduction program without exercise, the weight/fat will be harder to keep off.

Your weight/fat reduction program should contain these features:

1. It should be geared toward reducing body fat rather than simply shedding pounds.

2. It should *not* waste muscle, as many do. It should build muscle.

3. It should reduce weight gradually. Rapid weight loss throws the body into a starvation state, which is defensive and *fat-preserving.*

4. Focus on five to seven smaller meals a day. This regulates blood sugar and metabolism more evenly. Vow to no longer eat "three square meals a day."

5. Do not restrict calories. The average adult needs roughly 2,000 calories a day just to maintain basal metabolic rate. This sustains all the basic functions. If you increase your physical activity, which you will if you exercise, the caloric requirement *increases.* A diet that restricts calories will do two things. It will cause your body to metabolize its own muscle tissue in order to get the needed protein, and it will

conserve *fat* believing it is in a starvation state. Obviously, you want neither of these.

If you increase calories, how do you avoid becoming fatter? The answer is you modify the kind of calories you ingest.

Whatever program you choose to reduce your weight and body fat, it should contain exercise as a central component. If you take anything away from reading this section it should be this: *Muscle is the engine that burns the fuel of the body to generate energy.* Overweight/underlean people do not burn fat as well as fit people, so the activity must be geared toward more efficiently burning fat. This means both aerobic exercise *and* weight-lifting exercise to increase muscle mass.

"Why weight lifting?" Weight lifting builds muscles. When a heavy load is placed on the muscles, they burn the sugar glucose, an instant source of fuel. Weight lifting does not typically burn fat. It is an intense, concentrated activity that needs a quick supply of energy. However, muscles that have been trained through weight lifting become more efficient at burning fat during aerobic activity where the exercise is more sustained over a period of time. Thus, strong muscles means:

- More efficient burning of glucose during short bursts of activity.
- More efficient burning of fat during longer, aerobic activity. It also means more efficient burning of fat in general.

If you are intimidated by the prospect of lifting weights, you may take some comfort in the fact that men over age 65, with no previous experience with weights, are able to substantially increase their muscle mass by lifting weights in only six weeks. You can do the same. Just make sure your program is supervised by someone knowledgeable in the field and that it is tailored to your existing level of fitness.

Your aerobic program, which may consist of walking, bicycling, or one of several other types of exercise, should consist of 60-minute sessions and should be done five days a week. You may not be able to begin with 60 minutes. Start at five or ten and gradually work your way up to 60 over time. Twenty minutes of sustained exercise per day should be your absolute minimum.

Be patient and diligent, and realize that you are in this for the long haul. Don't expect to drop ten or fifteen pounds per week. One, two, or three might be more reasonable. The key should be, do you feel better and have more energy?

In Review

1. Being overweight or underlean (excessive body fat) can contribute to chronic fatigue.

2. The average person can benefit by keeping their body fat within an established range; 14–18 percent for men, 19–23 percent for women.

3. Many common weight-loss programs do not cause fat to be lost. Moreover, many encourage muscle wasting—exactly the opposite of what you want.

4. Your efforts to enhance your lean body mass, i.e., to increase your muscle-to-fat ratio, should include dietary management and exercise.

5. Dietary programs should be aimed at *fat* reduction and ideally involve detoxification support to assist in metabolizing the toxins that are liberated from fat during fat-loss.

6. Decrease consumption of saturated fat and trans fatty acids.

7. Decrease consumption of simple sugars.

8. Increase consumption (if you are not already doing so) of omega-3 fatty acids, monounsaturated fats, and complex carbohydrates.

9. Exercise should include both aerobic activity and weight lifting. This ensures that the muscles will be more efficient at burning both sugar and fat.

Chapter 8

Thyroid and Adrenal Problems

THYROID PROBLEMS HAVE long been recognized as an important cause of fatigue. When thyroid function becomes sluggish (hypothyroidism), you may experience fatigue, weakness, sluggishness, memory loss, skin problems, weight gain, joint aches, muscle cramps, infections, intolerance to cold, mood and personality changes such as depression, and other symptoms.

When thyroid function speeds up (hyperthyroidism), you may experience fatigue, insomnia, rapid or irregular heart beat, nervousness, anxiety, muscle weakness, weight loss, difficulty concentrating, intolerance to heat, and other symptoms. Notice that both *hypo*thyroidism and *hyper*thyroidism can produce symptoms of fatigue.

The thyroid gland combines iodine with the amino acid tyrosine to form thyroid hormone. Tetraiodothyronine (T4) is the inactive form of thyroid hormone. In order for the hormone to be activated, one atom of iodine must be removed to form triiodothyronine, or T3. This step of removing one atom of iodine depends on an enzyme called deiodinase, which itself is dependent on the trace element selenium.

The thyroid is important in many bodily functions such as:

- Protein synthesis
- Growth

- Temperature regulation
- Oxygen consumption of cells
- Metabolic rate

There are four basic considerations when thyroid function is found to be abnormal. They are:

- Insufficiency or deficiency of nutrients
- Toxicity
- Autoimmune reactions
- Trauma or injury

Insufficiency or deficiency. Nutrient insufficiency may cause the thyroid to produce inadequate amounts of thyroid hormone. Insufficiency may also create inefficient conversion of the inactive form of thyroid hormone to the active form. For example, selenium deficiency can cause the inactive T4 to be inefficiently converted to the active thyroid hormone T3.

Some doctors who treat thyroid problems may not give adequate consideration to the importance of nutrients in thyroid function. Prescribing thyroid drugs is often not enough to adequately regulate thyroid function. Below is just a brief summary of nutrients that influence thyroid function.[1]

Pyridoxine (B$_6$)	Riboflavin (B$_2$)
Niacin (B$_3$)	Vitamin A
Zinc	Copper
Chromium	Vitamin E
Cobalamin (B$_{12}$)	Vitamin C
Selenium	Tyrosine
Iodine	

Iodine is among the most important limiting factors in thyroid dysfunction. This nutrient is deficient in the soil of many regions of the country, especially the Midwest. For this reason, iodine was added to salt (iodized salt). However, some people may still not get enough iodine and may benefit from supplementation with this nutrient.

Excess iodine intake can also adversely effect thyroid function.

Low thyroid function also affects immune function. Lowered immune function can lead to repeated infections, which can be another cause of chronic fatigue. If you suffer from chronic infections and just seem to "catch" everything that goes around, consider having your thyroid function tested.

Toxicity. The thyroid is acutely sensitive to toxic chemicals that it encounters through food, air, and water. Fluoride is a thyroid toxin. Benzene, toluene, and other chemical substances to which we might be exposed interfere with normal thyroid function. Ingestion of alcohol or drugs (recreational or prescription), or autointoxication due to intestinal dysbiosis, may also impact thyroid function.

Chlorinated compounds are well known for their effects on thyroid function. Many of these compete directly with thyroid hormones or proteins that carry thyroid hormones. One such chemical, pentachlorophenol (used as a wood and leather preservative), was found to significantly lower the level of both the active and inactive form of thyroid hormone.[2] Moreover, thyroid hormone seemed to act as a carrier that allowed pentachlorophenol to enter the brain. How common might this be as a cause of poor thyroid function? No one is certain. However, one team of scientists found pentachlorophenol in the urine of 71 percent of people tested.[3]

Autoimmune reactions. Various factors can cause the immune system to attack its own organs, glands, joints, and other tissues. In essence, the immune system becomes less able to recognize self from non-self. This is called an autoimmune reaction. Infection of the intestinal tract by parasites or yeast can trigger an autoimmune thyroiditis. Viral infection, for example by the Epstein-Barr virus (EBV) associated with mononucleosis, can trigger an immune reaction that causes the body to turn on itself. In the case of EBV, the immune cells manufacture antibodies that are unleashed on the thyroid gland. Once the antibodies attack the thyroid gland, thyroid function begins to suffer, resulting in sluggishness, fatigue, lethargy, lowered body temperature, and depression. Intestinal dysbiosis can increase the likelihood of autoimmune reactions.

Trauma or injury. There is a recent hypothesis that trauma to the neck can trigger the development of thyroid problems. Keith Sehnert, M.D., of Minneapolis has encountered a number of patients whose thyroid problems began following an automobile accident or some other form of trauma. The trauma usually resulted in a cervical acceleration-deceleration injury (CAD), commonly known as whiplash. Sehnert has now followed more than 100 cases with careful histories and blood tests and has found what appears to be a significant correlation.[4] Time will tell if this proves to be true. However, if you have developed some symptoms of thyroid dysfunction and were in an accident within months of the onset of symptoms, you may wish to make this known to your chiropractic or medical physician.

Signs and Symptoms

Hypothyroidism[5]

Fatigue/lethargy
Weakness
Dry or rough skin or hair
Intolerance to cold
Depression
Difficulty concentrating
Puffy hands or face
Loss of outer third of
  eyebrow

Husky voice
Weight gain (often despite loss
  of appetite)
Joint aches, muscle cramps
Shortness of breath
Slow heart rate
Constipation
Mood or personality changes

Hyperthyroidism[6]

Nervousness/anxiety
Fatigue
Emotional instability
Muscle weakness
Muscle tremors
Rapid or irregular heartbeat
Perspiration
Intolerance to heat

Increased bowel movements
Weight loss (often despite
  increased appetite)
Difficulty concentrating
Menstrual irregularities
Eye irritation or protruding
  eyes
Thyroid swelling or tenderness in the lower neck

Laboratory Tests

Thyroid Function Panel that includes:

- T3 resin uptake
- Free T4 Index
- TSH (thyroid stimulating hormone)
- FAMA (fluorescent-activated microsphere assay, or thyroid antibody panel)

Thyroid function tests are sometimes normal even in the presence of thyroid dysfunction. One method of determining if your thyroid function is low is to take your temperature under the armpit each morning. The basal temperature test is performed as follows: Shake down a thermometer before going to bed at night and leave it on the nightstand. Immediately upon waking in the morning (before rising from bed), place the thermometer in the axilla. Lie still for ten minutes. After ten minutes remove the thermometer and check the reading. A reading below 97.8 degrees F suggests low thyroid function. The test should be done on at least three consecutive days. Women should take the test while not menstruating.

Some say the axillary temperature test is more an indicator of basal metabolism and is not specific for thyroid problems. This may well be true. Consider that for every one degree Fahrenheit you raise your body temperature you increase your metabolic rate, e.g. energy, by 13 percent. So, if your temperature is low, you might do well to find out why and take steps to correct it.

Neither the axillary temperature nor the thyroid blood tests are foolproof, but abnormalities in either, coupled with the classic symptoms, should cause suspicion.

Treatment

Oral therapy with synthetic thyroid hormone is the most common treatment for hypothyroidism. Some doctors believe that synthetic thyroid hormone is not as effective as desiccated thyroid tissue. Other doctors prescribe nutrients in addition to desiccated thyroid tissue.

Management of thyroid problems using nutrition alone can be helpful, but often requires augmentation with thyroid tissue or medication. Addressing gastrointestinal problems and chemical toxicity is also important.

In some fatigued patients, thyroid problems overlap adrenal problems. In these cases, the status of the adrenal glands and the thyroid gland must be assessed. The appropriate treatment should be undertaken only after this determination is made.

Sluggish Adrenal Glands

The adrenal glands rest atop the kidneys and are an integral part of the endocrine system. They are responsible for producing several important hormones and are critical to the stress response. One of the most prominent signs of adrenal gland insufficiency is chronic fatigue.

As a response to stress, the adrenal glands produce DHEA (dehydroepiandrosterone) and cortisol. Both hormones have predictable effects on body chemistry. In health, the ratio of the two is optimal. The hypothalamus and pituitary gland, both in the brain, are sensitive to the amount of cortisol circulating in the blood. When cortisol reaches a certain level, the hypothalamus and pituitary modify production of adrenal hormones. This system of checks and balances ensures that hormone levels are properly regulated. However, certain factors may overload this system.

During chronic stress, excess cortisol is often produced. Moreover, the hypothalamus and pituitary gland may grow less sensitive to the changes and do not turn off production of cortisol as they should. When this happens a series of problems may occur such as decreased immune function, altered blood sugar regulation, fat accumulation, and changes in behavior.

If chronic stress persists, more cortisol is produced, but less DHEA. As the amount of cortisol becomes higher while DHEA becomes lower, the adverse health consequences grow.[7] Meanwhile, excess epinephrine (adrenalin) is produced, which has it's own set of adverse consequences.

The adrenal glands produce their array of hormones in a complex symphony that is orchestrated by two structures in the brain called the hypothalamus and the pituitary gland. When stress and poor nutrition lead to altered hormone levels, imbalance in endocrine function can lead to substantial fatigue. The only road back appears to be stress management coupled with appropriate biochemical therapy.

The kinds of stressors that tax the adrenal glands include many of those already discussed in this book such as:

Physical trauma	Chemical toxins
Poor diet	Excess exercise
Lack of sleep	Infections
Emotional trauma	Anxiety, depression
Prescription drugs	Pregnancy

When problems of adrenal insufficiency are identified and corrected, the effect on energy, stamina, and vitality can be substantial.

Signs and Symptoms

Fatigue	Nervousness
Irritability	Depression
Inability to concentrate	Weakness
Frustration	Lightheadedness
Insomnia	Premenstrual tension
Sweet cravings	Headaches
Allergies	Scanty perspiration

Laboratory Tests

- Salivary cortisol. Measured at 8 A.M., 12 P.M., 4 P.M., and 11 P.M.

- Salivary DHEA (dehydroepiandrosterone)

- Postural blood pressure. This is taken first lying down, then retaken upon standing. If blood pressure falls upon standing, adrenal insufficiency may exist.

Treatment

Adrenal problems that are not serious or life-threatening are often treated with a combination of low doses of cortisol, DHEA, various herbs, and nutrients. Each of these is used under very specific circumstances and this is determined by laboratory tests. When the specific stage of adrenal insufficiency is determined, the result of treatment can be very rewarding.

It is important to recognize that treatment with excessive levels of cortisol can suppress immune function, damage tissue, and alter the inflammatory process. Doctors who treat adrenal insufficiency with cortisol use very tiny amounts—usually sufficient to stimulate adrenal gland function. These are called physiologic doses as opposed to therapeutic doses. DHEA is used with similar caution. Many doctors who use DHEA therapeutically feel that doses should never exceed 40 mg per day.[8] When used properly under the right conditions, DHEA is an important means of improving hormone regulation and improving energy.

Nutrients important in adrenal gland function include pantothenic acid, vitamin C, serine phosphatides, and pyridoxine. Botanicals sometimes used to help restore adrenal function include ginseng, licorice, and gotukola. This is a complex area of treatment and should only be undertaken after a careful assessment of hormone levels. Doctors who attempt to treat adrenal insufficiency without getting a careful picture of hormone levels may be doing their patients a disservice.

Stress management *must* be a component of any effort to balance adrenal gland function. Even the best laid biochemical and nutritional strategies may fail if some form of stress management is not undertaken. These programs come in many shapes and sizes, but usually include such things as exercise, deep breathing, visualization, imagery work, biofeedback, counseling, chi gong, and meditation.

In Review

1. Poor thyroid function (overactive or underactive) is an important cause of fatigue.

2. Poor thyroid function can contribute to lowered immunity, which makes one more susceptible to bacterial and viral infection—also causes of fatigue.

3. The thyroid is highly dependent upon adequate nutrition. Any thyroid treatment should include nutritional support and not just thyroid hormone replacement.

4. Many environmental substances can impair thyroid function. Toxicity should be considered with thyroid disorders.

5. Adrenal insufficiency can cause fatigue.

6. The hormones cortisol and DHEA can be measured in saliva to assess adrenal function.

7. A combination of cortisol, DHEA, herbs, and nutrients is being used by some doctors to restore adrenal function.

Chapter 9

The Fitness Factor:
The Paradox of Inactivity and Energy

LACK OF ADEQUATE physical activity and poor physical fitness are common causes of fatigue and low vitality. It may seem paradoxical that exercise, which makes one tired, would improve symptoms of tiredness and fatigue. However, there is little doubt that exercise improves overall energy. For example, almost all people with a condition called fibromyalgia suffer from chronic fatigue. In one study, 83 percent of those with fibromyalgia were not engaging in regular exercise, and 65 percent were well below average in aerobic fitness.[1] Those with poor aerobic fitness are considered more likely to develop this painful muscle condition than those who exercise regularly. Moreover, exercise has proven helpful in relieving the pain and fatigue of fibromyalgia.

Physical activity and movement are vital to maintaining health. They increase muscle mass, increase oxygenation of the cells, promote the elimination of toxins through sweating, move waste products through the lymphatic vessels, help return used blood through the veins (which have no muscles or pump of their own), stimulate immune function, improve memory and cognitive function, strengthen bones, improve bowel function, speed the burning of fat, and many other functions.

How Exercise Improves Energy

    Increases muscle mass (the engine of metabolism)
    Reduces body fat
    Increases pumping volume of the heart
    Improves circulation
    Improves blood sugar regulation
    Lowers blood fats
    Improves mood
    Improves mental capacity

Many of the causes of fatigue listed elsewhere in this book can also be improved with exercise. These include:

Diabetes	Hypoglycemia
Overweight/underlean	Elevated blood fats
Sleep difficulty	Fibromyalgia
Depression	Heart disease (certain types)

Physical activity is one of the most important things you can do to improve your energy. Of all the factors described in this book to help you improve your energy, movement may be the most straightforward. It doesn't require any fancy lab tests, drugs, supplements, diets, or protocols. It merely requires your commitment, diligence, and effort.

Unfortunately, the physical activity of Americans seems to be declining. According to the President's Council on Physical Fitness and Sports, roughly 60 percent of Americans are sedentary. When asked why they did not exercise, the sedentary folk reported being "too tired, too busy, and too lazy to exercise." Sixty-four percent reported that they would like to exercise more but didn't have the time. However, 84 percent reported watching at least several hours of television a week.[2]

You don't have to do intense aerobics for two hours nor must you throw around free-weights with the behemoths at the gym six days a week. Exercise means moving your muscles, expanding your lungs, sweating, and toning your body. It should be a combination of aerobic conditioning exercises and weight-bearing muscle-building exercises. Why the two? The term aerobic means "with oxygen." It is usually used to describe activity that uses or requires oxygen. Aerobic exercise increases oxygen to the tissues and improves overall metabolism. With thorough oxygen delivery to the tissues one generally has more energy. Weight-bearing exercises, some of which are anaerobic, or without oxygen, build muscle size. Remember, muscle is the engine that drives energy metabolism. The more muscle you have (to a point, as long as aerobic fitness is maintained), the better able you are to burn fat and sugar to produce energy.

Recall from chapter 1 the description of mitochondria, the little power-packed structures within your cells that produce energy. When people don't exercise, the number of mitochondria in the cells actually goes down. When you exercise, the number goes up. It is also very specific. The number of mitochondria only increase in the specific muscle groups that are being exercised. Those people who have more mitochondria are more able to produce energy on demand. Those with numerous and more active mitochondria are also better at burning fat as a source of fuel.[3]

This is an important key to keep in mind. Muscles have the advantage of burning two forms of fuel: sugar and fat. For quick bursts of energy such as lifting weights, the body needs a quick source of fuel. Sugar fits the bill. For longer bouts of exercise, the body burns fat. People who are physically unfit (who often have too much body fat) are inefficient at burning fat. They burn sugar just fine, but their fat-burning ability is poor.

In fact, when the unfit or overfat person exercises, sugar is rapidly used up, causing a drop in blood sugar. This leads to hunger for sweets. If sweets are eaten, they tend to be converted into fat. If this urge is ignored and nothing is eaten, the body uses the protein from muscle as a source of fuel. This can lead to an actual wasting of muscle and can decrease lean body mass. In order to improve their fat-burning ability, the unfit or overfat person should consider both weight lifting and aerobic fitness activity.

Various forms of movement have been used to help patients who are chronically tired or who suffer from chronic fatigue. Below are some common exercises that can help improve your general fitness:

Stair stepping	Stair climbing
Bicycling	Jumping rope
Cross country skiing	Jogging
Walking	Swimming
Treadmill	Aerobic dance
Basketball	Hiking
Racquetball	Skating (roller or ice)
Soccer	Tennis
Chopping wood	Weight training
Sit ups	Push ups
Chin ups	Rowing
Yoga	T'ai Chi

Signs and Symptoms

The signs and symptoms of poor physical fitness are very general. There is no specific medical condition or set of symptoms associated with physical inactivity. Physical inactivity seems to affect many body systems simultaneously. Some common manifestations are listed below:

Chronic fatigue and low vitality
Poor sleep or insomnia
Shortness of breath on exertion
Chronic health problems
Weak muscles
Mood swings
Aching muscles after minimal exertion
Easily injured during strenuous activity

Laboratory Tests

There are no commonly used laboratory tests used to assess physical inactivity. Obviously, you know whether or not you are physically active. However, some fitness experts use body fat analysis, respiratory volume, and various other indicators to determine the baseline level of fitness. These are informative and give an indication of current status, but they are not essential. An advantage of these analyses is they give you a baseline against which to gauge your improvement. For example, if your body fat is measured at 35 percent you can be assured that your fitness level is low, that there are increased demands on your heart, that you do not burn calories as efficiently as you should, and that you are at risk to a variety of ills.

Treatment

The solution to fatigue that is related to insufficient physical activity is to become physically active.

If you have never been physically active, there is a certain amount of emotional inertia you may encounter. One way to overcome this inertia is to see yourself as a physically fit person. Do not view yourself as one who couldn't do this or that in years past. Look at yourself as physically vibrant. Change your beliefs about what you are capable of. Everyone is an athlete. The only difference between those who are doing it and those who are not is desire, attitude, and action.

When you begin a fitness program, keep a few things in mind:

1. Always tailor your workout to your existing level of fitness. I have seen far too many patients excited about exercising go out and push too hard at the outset. The next day, or in some cases for the next week, their muscles are sore, they feel sick, and some feel as though they have the flu. This is much like an overtraining syndrome. Begin your training gradually.

2. Have a physical before you begin training, especially if you have an existing medical condition. If you suffer from chronic fatigue syndrome, fibromyalgia, diabetes, heart disease, or another medical condition, consult your doctor before beginning an exercise program. Exercise must be tailored very specifically in these cases.

3. Exercise with someone who is in about the same shape as yourself. Otherwise you may get discouraged.

4. Make sure your exercise is FUN. If it isn't fun you won't continue for long.

5. Vary your routines. You may wish to ride a bicycle or exercycle three times a week and swim twice a week. You may want to walk

three miles a day every other day and lift weights the other days. Variation keeps you from getting bored.

6. Try to get involved with a program that adds a social atmosphere to your exercise. Exercising in solitude takes a lot of discipline. Even elite athletes prefer to exercise and train with other people.

7. If you are uncertain about where to begin, consult a fitness trainer who can help you tailor a program to your specific needs.

8. Consume adequate antioxidant nutrients that protect against the free-radical effects of exercise. Included are vitamin E, vitamin C, beta-carotene, selenium, glutathione, and coenzyme Q_{10}.

A note of caution is in order for those who suffer from chronic fatigue *syndrome*. Many who suffer from this experience an alteration in energy metabolism that makes symptoms worse. This is a poorly understood phenomenon, but has been well documented. If you suffer from CFS, it is especially important that you begin your exercise under the supervision of a doctor.

In Review

1. Physical inactivity can lead to tiredness, fatigue, low vitality, sluggish immunity, and a host of other ills.

2. Engaging in physical activity should be a routine part of one's daily life.

3. The activity should be pleasurable, but challenging.

4. The activity should be tailored to your individual level of fitness. Excessive physical activity for a sedentary person only leads to frustration, injury, or altered immunity. Gradually increase your exercise intensity as your fitness level improves.

5. Vary your exercise routines.

6. Eat well. Cliff Sheat's book *Lean Bodies* is an excellent guide to reducing body fat and building muscle.

Chapter 10

The Athlete with Fatigue:
The Cost of Overexertion

AN ATHLETE IS ANYONE who engages in physical activity or sport that requires physical exertion, skill, balance, strength, endurance, and stamina. Whether you jog, bicycle, work out at the gym four times a week, compete in occasional amateur events, or compete at the collegiate, international, or professional level, this chapter is about you. The athletes most likely to suffer from fatigue as a result of their training or sport are generally those who engage in more strenuous activity. For example, a distance runner is more likely to suffer from sport-related fatigue than a bowler. We commonly see fatigue in average people who simply train hard and overlook certain key elements.

What is fatigue in athletes? By fatigue I mean:

- A general feeling of tiredness or lack of energy during the day
- Declining or poor performance
- Fatigue during exercise
- Slow recovery after exercise

There are several reasons that athletes are susceptible to suffering from fatigue. Most of these causes are preventable and require some basic knowledge and preparation. Others come with the territory, but can be overcome with nutrition and common sense.

There are seven basic factors that contribute to fatigue in athletes at all levels:

1. Heavy training may normally suppress immunity and increase susceptibility to viral and bacterial infection.

2. Inadequate fluid intake and dehydration lead to fatigue.

3. Poor nutrition and unbalanced diets lead to poor energy production.

4. Inadequate rest harms immunity, slows exercise recovery, and can prevent muscle building.

5. Overtraining contributes to lowered immunity, poor recovery, and fatigue.

6. Exposure to environmental pollutants during training affects oxygen exchange and energy production.

7. Training can lead to nutrient loss.

Almost all of these can be overcome with proper training techniques, dietary habits, and nutritional supplementation. Let's briefly look at each of the above areas and see why they contribute to fatigue.

Training Suppresses Immunity. There is a paradox about athletic training in that it can both stimulate and suppress immunity. When women with susceptibility to upper respiratory infection began a program of 45 minutes of walking each day, their symptoms improved and immune parameters improved.[1] Yet, sedentary subjects who were placed in an intense aerobic training course (45 minutes a day, five days a week for 15 weeks) suffered *decreased* immunity and increased infection susceptibility.[2] The difference between the two studies is that in the first study, moderate exercise was undertaken that matched the level of fitness. In the second study, the level of physical exertion greatly exceeded the people's capability and fitness level. When the athlete's level of training is matched with his or her level of fitness, immune function actually improves.[3]

The results of many studies on athletic training and immune suppression are convincing. A few are noted below:

- Athletes are more susceptible to bacterial infections.[4]
- Elite swimmers are more susceptible to infections as the season progresses.[5]
- In 530 runners followed for one year, infections were related to weekly mileage.[6]
- Runners were twice as likely to suffer upper respiratory infections following a race.[7]
- Distance runners lose more training days to infection than to injury.[8]

The issue of infection and athletes is of great importance. Fifty-two elite American athletes missed the 1992 Olympics because of infection.[9] Many more competed poorly because of lowered immunity. Sprinter Carl Lewis, one of the fastest 100-meter runners in the world, failed to make the Olympic team because of a viral infection during the Olympic trials. When the Olympics were finally held months later, he was inserted as the anchor on the 4 X 100 relay team and ran the fastest 100-meter leg in history. Many athletes competing in the 1994 winter games in Lillehammer, Norway, were slowed by infections. Some missed qualifying because of infections.

All of this does not mean we should avoid exercise or that athletic training is inherently bad. Indeed, when properly done, athletic training improves immune function. The way to optimize the effects of training so that immune function is bolstered rather than suppressed is to:

1. Avoid overtraining.
2. Tailor your workouts to your level of fitness.
3. Get adequate rest.
4. Consume adequate calories and avoid junk food.
5. Avoid training when you suffer from a cold or flu.
6. Optimize your antioxidant nutrient status.

Whenever you exercise, your body generates free radicals. Free radicals are highly reactive chemical species that can cause chain reactions in cell tissue. Free-radical production is one reason for the muscle soreness that follows exercise and for the decline in immune function that may follow exercise. Antioxidant nutrients such as vitamin C, vitamin E, beta-carotene, glutathione, selenium, coenzyme Q_{10}, and others help to quench (or put out the fire of) free radicals, thus preventing the damage they might do. Adequate stores of antioxidant nutrients such as these can therefore protect against the damaging effects of free radicals released during exercise.

A group of 92 marathon runners was placed on either a vitamin C supplement or a placebo for three weeks prior to a race. Of those taking the placebo, 68 percent showed signs and symptoms consistent with upper respiratory infection, while only 33 percent of those on vitamin C showed such signs.[10] In another study, researchers found that vitamin E supplementation reduced the oxidative damage that occurs with exercise.[11]

Nutrients important in reducing the oxidative damage and immune-suppressive effects of exercise include: vitamin C, vitamin E, beta-carotene, glutathione, N-acetylcysteine, selenium, and coenzyme Q_{10}.

Inadequate Fluid Intake and Dehydration. Fluid loss is a common reason for fatigue in athletes. Whenever you exercise your body temperature rises. As temperature rises, the body perspires in an attempt to cool itself, which leads to fluid loss. In a two-hour period of intense exercise, a person may lose five to eight pounds of fluid. For every pound of water lost, there is a significant drop in the efficiency with which the body produces energy. Performance also suffers when water is lost. In fact, well-hydrated athletes almost always perform better than comparable but poorly hydrated athletes.

The body's thirst sensors are not highly sensitive during exercise, so thirst is not a good indicator of the need for water. In order for the athlete to consume adequate fluid, he or she must consume a regular amount of fluid during each hour of training. Otherwise, dehydration, low performance, and fatigue may set in.

Another important reason to drink fluid during exercise is to replace carbohydrates. Whenever body temperature goes up, the body uses more glycogen, which is the stored form of sugar used for fuel during physical activity. It is one fuel that makes the muscles run (fat is the other). As you exercise, glycogen is burned in the muscles, which depletes the stores in your body. These stores must be replaced and the muscles must be supplied with an ongoing source of glycogen to sustain an endurance-type activity—cycling or running, for example. In order to store glycogen, the body requires significant amounts of water.

Other substances lost during the perspiration of heavy training (that also affect fatigability) are electrolytes like magnesium and potassium. These are important to muscle function (not to mention heart muscle function). Recall from the chapter on nutrients that magnesium deficiency is commonly associated with fatigue states. If you are working out and not replacing magnesium, chances are good that your body has insufficient magnesium to function at its peak and that your fatigue may be helped by magnesium supplementation.

So, to prevent dehydration (and thus fatigue) the athlete should consider replenishing with three basic substances during and after training sessions:

- *Fluid.* Water is the best source of fluid.

- *Carbohydrate.* A five to seven percent mixture of polymerized glucose plus fructose is considered by many to be the best means to replenish carbohydrate during and after exercise.[12] It is used by many Olympic and professional athletes. Avoid sucrose-based drinks that are so common in the marketplace. Sugared carbonated beverages are ill-advised as well.

- *Electrolytes.* This should include potassium, magnesium, chromium, phosphate, and sodium.

There are numerous rehydration formulas on the market and there are sure to be more. Dr. Michael Colgan, who works with many world-class athletes, suggests Hydra Fuel by Twin Labs. Others who work with Olympic athletes use Endura by Metagenics.

If you are in any kind of regular workout program, a fluid replacement supplement such as those above (to be used during workouts) should be a regular part of your training regimen. After workouts continue to drink extra water for six to twelve hours.

Poor Nutrition and Unbalanced Diets. Athletes are notorious for their pursuit of performance-enhancing diets, nutrients, and drugs. There is a constant search to raise one's level of performance or exceed that of a competitor. Elite athletes, high school athletes, and weekend warriors are no different in this regard. Because of this, many embark on ill-advised programs that do not support them nutritionally. The result may be fatigability.

For example, wrestlers commonly cut calories in an effort to "make weight." This often leads to dehydration, poor kidney function, and poor nutrient intake. In one study of wrestlers, most consumed less than the RDA for protein, vitamins A, B_1, and B_6, iron, zinc, and magnesium.

Chronic fatigue symptoms are common in dancers and gymnasts. In one study, dancers and gymnasts were found to consume less than the RDA for vitamin B_6, folic acid, calcium, zinc, and magnesium.[13] The nutritional and metabolic status of young female gymnasts is poor because of efforts to remain lean and small for competition. Young gymnasts often consume inadequate calories, inadequate protein, are nutrient-deficient, and have inadequate body fat stores. Estrogen, progesterone, and growth hormone production become disrupted. This leads to poor growth and development and can leave lasting metabolic and psychological scars. In some reports, the bone density of young female gymnasts has been comparable to that of an 80-year-old woman. Any coach, parent, or athlete associated with gymnastics must take great care to ensure that optimum nutritional guidelines are followed.

In another study, female long-distance runners were low in iron, zinc, copper, magnesium, and other nutrients, and only consumed a fraction of the calories needed to keep up that kind of physical activity.[14]

Athletes also commonly overemphasize protein and sugar at the expense of complex carbohydrates. Poor muscle glycogen stores may result when training is heavy. This is especially true in endurance sports. The average person needs roughly 2,000 calories per day to meet basic requirements. It is estimated that cyclists in the Tour de France required up to 8,000 k/cal per day to replace energy expenditure.[15] Those who do not consume this much usually fail to compete or drop out. Complex carbohydrates must be emphasized over snack bars as a source of energy. While complex carbohydrates are important in general training regimens, simple carbohydrates are acceptable immediately following training sessions or competition.

Runners often do not get adequate fat to meet their energy needs. It is not uncommon for a runner to have a body fat of nine percent and a daily fat intake of only 10 percent of total calories. This is not enough to meet the endurance needs of the athlete. The quality of fat is critical here. Saturated fat and trans fatty acids are not good sources.

Rapid weight loss can present nutrition and fluid problems. Athletes such as wrestlers who attempt to lose weight quickly must be aware of the dangers. All efforts to lose weight should be carried out during periods of light training and should be *avoided* during times when competition is planned.[16]

If you are serious about training, whether you are training for competition or just want to stay in shape, it would be wise to consult a nutrition-oriented professional who is familiar with the specific needs of your sport.

Sleep and Rest. Adequate sleep and rest are critical to overcoming or preventing fatigue. After just a few days of inadequate sleep, your immune function begins to decline. Your reaction time and clarity of thinking also suffer measurably. Sustained periods of insufficient sleep take a more lasting toll. Athletes, who are placing much greater physical demands on their bodies than the average person, *must* ensure they get adequate sleep or the body will simply not regenerate and repair itself. Athletes who do not get at least eight or nine hours of sleep a day will gradually run themselves down. The result will be lowered performance, slower recovery after events or training sessions, injuries, and fatigability. Also, any time you increase your training intensity, you must also increase the amount of rest you get.[17]

Overtraining. Overtraining occurs when you have exceeded your body's limits. This takes into consideration your level of fitness, the amount of rest you receive, the number of hours per day you exercise, your nutritional status, your diet, your age, your percentage body fat, and any existing medical conditions you may have. According to Dr. Michael Colgan, author of *Optimum Sports Nutrition*, any time you increase your level of training by 10 percent over previous levels you will experience a downturn in immune function. For example, a runner who typically runs five miles per day and decides to abruptly add another mile (or 20 percent) to his schedule may possibly experience a drop in immune function. Overtraining also comes about by combining a nutritionally inadequate diet with heavy workouts and inadequate rest (or sleep).

Dr. Colgan's strategy to identify overtraining is as follows:

1. *Waking Pulse Rate.* Athletes should grow accustomed to taking their waking pulse rate each morning before rising. The pulse of a well-trained athlete will be between 40 and 60 beats per minute. If the baseline rate increases by more than 8–10 beats per minute, it should be taken as a warning that illness or overtraining may be present.[18] In such cases, a reduction in training or increase in rest may be advised. A doctor should be seen to check for illness.

2. *Waking Weight.* Waking weight should never drop more than three pounds. In such cases, reduction in training and increased rest may be advised.

3. *Insomnia.* Sudden onset of insomnia may signal overtraining or illness. Sudden insomnia often leads to decrease in immune function.

4. *Poor Recovery.* Fatigued athletes may experience an unusually high pulse rate during exercise with a slower return to normalcy.[19]

Summary of Signs of Overtraining

Slow recovery
Poor performance, feeling trapped in a routine
Loss of purpose, energy, and competitive drive

Fatigue during exercise and rest
Insomnia, loss of appetite, excessive sweating
Increased susceptibility to infections
Anxiety, irritability, emotional liability
Loss of libido
Muscle pain

Exposure to Environmental Pollutants. Athletes in certain sports are more likely to be exposed to chemicals that not only interfere with performance, but also affect liver function, muscle function, and reduce antioxidant nutrient stores in the body.

For example, competitive swimmers suffer inordinately from asthma. They also become more susceptible to infection as the season progresses. In one study, 92 percent of 251 competitive swimmers had symptoms of respiratory distress. Roughly three fourths of those with asthma were diagnosed *after* they began swimming.

One important contributor is continued exposure to chloride from swimming pools. Chloride is a powerful oxidant that interacts with lung tissue, leading to inflammation and mucus formation. Chloroform, a byproduct of chlorination, is present in indoor swimming pools due to the use of sodium hypochlorite. In a study of 127 people, researchers compared the level of chloroform in the blood of people who swam every day, a few days a week, and who were merely in the pool area. Those who swam most frequently during the week had higher blood levels of chloroform.[20] Anyone who swims regularly must receive additional antioxidants on a daily basis, with greater doses during training or before competition. I've found this to be helpful in swimmers with and without asthma.

Runners and cyclists who train in city environments are at risk to increased exposure to aromatic hydrocarbons, nitrogen oxides, sulfur dioxide, carbon monoxide, ozone, and other potent oxidants present in smog and automobile exhaust. For example, runners training in Central Park in New York City experienced a three-fold increase in carbon monoxide levels in their blood (measured as carboxyhemoglobin). This was twice the increase experienced by people merely standing in Central Park.[21] Carbon monoxide binds tightly to the hemoglobin molecule in red blood cells (which is the main oxygen transporter in the body) and prevents the transport of oxygen to body tissues. The result of too little oxygen is fatigue and listlessness. Anti-oxidant nutrient supplementation is essential in these athletes.

The following recommendations can help minimize the risks of exercising in air pollution:

- Schedule outdoor workouts in early morning or after sunset.
- If exercise is performed during rush hour, choose windy areas with little traffic.
- Breathe through the nose rather than the mouth to utilize filtration.
- Exercise indoors during any pollution alert.
- Avoid second-hand cigarette smoke before and after exercise.
- Take extra antioxidants.

Training and Nutrient Needs. The subject of sports nutrition is far too complex to discuss in depth here. You should recognize, however, that athletic training causes certain nutrients to be used more rapidly while others are lost through the sweat and urine. Rather than cover these in depth, I'll cite just a few of examples.

Adolescent athletes appear to be especially susceptible to developing iron deficiency. Iron deficiency in adolescents reduces performance, lengthens recovery times, increases infection susceptibility, and can cause fatigue. Deficiency occurs because of heavy training (especially among endurance athletes), poor diets, and blood loss through menstruation in girls. Heavy training causes loss of iron through sweating and red blood cell destruction. Adolescent athletes should have a serum ferritin test done. A diet history should also be evaluated to make sure that the diet contains adequate amounts of iron.

Other Nutritional Considerations

1. *Magnesium.* Magnesium loss in athletes is common.

2. *Iron.* Insufficiency isore common in athletes who restrict calories to control weight: gymnasts, dancers, wrestlers. One study of

female distance runners showed that 91 percent had inadequate iron in their diets. 80 percent of the females were iron-deficient, but not one of them showed hemoglobin levels below 12 g/dl.[22] Menstrual blood loss, pregnancy, and childbirth also tax iron stores. Total iron loss accompanying pregnancy, parturition, and lactation is nearly 900 mg. Iron status in the postpartum athlete should be carefully assessed.

Sweating does not appear to cause significant iron loss in athletes.[23] Gastrointestinal blood loss can occur in female athletes and long-distance runners, which may lead to anemia. Iron deficiency significant enough to cause anemia can have a substantial impact on work capacity, endurance, oxygen delivery, and muscle metabolism.

Athletes who suffer from chronic infections should not take iron until they have had their iron status checked. Athletes who are not iron-deficient or anemic but who supplement with iron may experience increased susceptibility to infection.

3. *Coenzyme Q_{10}.* CoQ_{10} appears to improve muscle function and protect against exercise-induced muscle injury.[24] CoQ_{10} also has an immunoregulatory effect on both cell-mediated and humoral immunity.

4. *Vitamin C.* Reduces the impact of free radicals generated during exercise and reduces the impact of free radicals to which athletes are exposed when training in smog or air-polluted areas. Vitamin C was recently shown to relieve delayed-onset muscle soreness in athletes. Muscle soreness was relieved in more than 75 percent of subjects, the observed range of relief being between 24 and 44 percent.[25] Vitamin C also increases several aspects of immune function. Vitamin C should be given as part of an antioxidant formula to all athletes.

5. *Taurine.* Useful in asthmatic swimmers constantly exposed to chlorine. Taurine is necessary to detoxify hypochlorite radicals. Taurine also helps regulate the transport of electrolytes such as potassium and magnesium in smooth muscle (including the heart).

6. *Beta-carotene.* Has a dose-dependent effect on immune function. Also acts as a potent free-radical scavenger. Beta-carotene can be given as part of a routine supplement in training.

7. *Zinc.* Significant amounts of zinc are lost through sweating. Zinc needs increase as iron and fat metabolism increase during exercise. Zinc is necessary for the action of the enzyme lactate dehydrogenase, which serves to metabolize lactic acid produced during muscle activity. There is evidence that athletes have poor zinc status as a result of training.[26] In a recent study of competitive athletes, 60 percent had zinc intake below the RDA despite supplementation.[27] Zinc deficiency also leads to altered immune function.

8. *Selenium.* An essential component of glutathione peroxidase and the antioxidant defense system.

9. *Vitamin E.* Vitamin E prevents the free-radical damage that normally occurs during exercise.[28] Vitamin E is important in preventing injury in athletes and in maintaining immune function.

10. *Glutamine.* This amino acid is an important energy source for lymphocytes and muscle cells. In one study, plasma glutamine levels were significantly lower in underperforming fatigued athletes.[29]

11. *Rehydration formula.* Water must be supplied before, during, and after exercise to prevent dehydration and its concomitant problems. Carbohydrates and electrolytes must also be supplied.

12. *Glutathione.* L-glutathione is one of the principal antioxidants in human tissue. It exists in amounts 100 times greater than vitamin C and is important in preventing free-radical damage of muscle associated with training or training in polluted environments. Glutathione can be severely depleted during heavy exercise. In one study, animals exercised to exhaustion experienced a 40 percent drop in muscle glutathione and an 80 percent drop in liver glutathione.[30] Glutathione is vital to the removal of heavy metals from tissue stores.

In Review

1. Athletes commonly suffer from fatigue.

2. The main reasons include the following: a) Training can suppress immunity and increase susceptibility to viral and bacterial infection. b) Inadequate fluid intake and dehydration. c) Overtraining contributes to lowered immunity and fatigue. d) Poor nutrition and unbalanced

diets lead to poor energy production. e) Inadequate rest harms immunity and slows exercise recovery. f) Exposure to environmental pollutants during training. g) Training can lead to nutrient loss.

3. Athletes should not abruptly increase their training level by more than ten percent at any given time.

4. Athletes should consume additional antioxidant nutrients to minimize the oxidative stress associated with heavy exercise.

5. Athletes should always consume extra fluids, carbohydrate, and electrolytes to replace that which is lost during training.

6. Nutritional supplementation can offset many of the rigors of training.

7. If you are an athlete who suffers from fatigue you may need to alter your training regimen.

8. If you suffer from infections or lowered immunity you may need to take time off training and improve your nutritional status in order to recover.

9. Rest and sleep are vitally important to prevention of fatigue and to recovery should you suffer from fatigue.

If you are serious about enhancing your performance and getting the facts on optimizing training through proper nutrition, I highly recommend you read the book *Optimum Sports Nutrition* by Dr. Michael Colgan (Advanced Research Press, New York, 1993).

Chapter 11

Posture and Body Mechanics

A LARGE PERCENTAGE of the energy produced in the human body goes toward maintaining the body in space. Muscles are continually contracting and relaxing, orchestrating the delicate movements that maintain our posture. This process is very energy-intensive. Yet it goes on almost completely without our knowledge. The human frame is designed to function with its various movements balanced over a specific center of gravity. The body expends the least amount of energy when balanced over this center. If the center of gravity shifts too far forward, backward, or sideward, the muscles must generate an enormous amount of energy to maintain the skeleton in space.

A growing number of doctors believe that poor body mechanics, poor posture, and altered center of gravity cause certain muscle groups to be in a state of excessive activity (hypertonicity). These muscles require substantial fuel and energy to maintain this for any length of time. When muscles are forced into this state of chronic contraction, they begin to produce chemical irritants that can cause pain. Moreover, such muscles become easily fatigued, which ultimately affects their ability to carry out their normal functions of energy metabolism. If this continues long enough and affects enough muscle groups (which it commonly does), the result may be generalized fatigue that impacts the entire body.

Most women are already familiar with the effect of body mechanics on energy. They just aren't aware of it. The culprit is high heels. After spending a day in high-heeled shoes, most women feel fatigued, worn out, bushed, and can't wait to get them off their feet. The higher the heels and the longer they're worn, the greater the fatigue. The reason for this is that high heels shift the center of gravity well forward from its normal position. The muscles of the calves, buttocks, back, and shoulders must work overtime in a futile attempt to shift the center of gravity back where it belongs. This constant muscle activity, called static loading, causes the buildup of lactic acid in muscles and reduces the amount of oxygen available to the tissues. It diminishes the elimination of toxins from the muscles and consumes much-needed ATP (recall the energy molecule from chapter 1). This often leaves women very fatigued.

The phenomenon of increased energy demand and high-heels has been studied and published in the *Journal of Orthopedics and Sports Physical Therapy*. Researchers found that high-heel wearers experienced increases in heart rate and oxygen consumption. Interestingly, oxygen consumption and heart rate increased with heel height. The authors advised that women should avoid wearing heels with a heel height greater than 5.08 cm (2 inches).[1] My experience with patients suggests that one- or two-inch heels are still high enough to produce fatigue and energy problems.

A similar problem occurs in those who are overweight. Your body is the heaviest thing most of you will ever lift, and it is lifted on a daily basis. Increasing the body weight by only 15 or 20 pounds places increased energy demands on the body's metabolism. If this extra weight is fat, the demands are even greater. As weight increases, there is almost always a shift in the center of gravity, depending upon where most of the weight is added.

The problem of poor body mechanics is in no way restricted to women or those who are overweight. It can affect anyone at any age and may be an important contributor to chronic fatigue in those affected.

In his book *Sitting on the Job*, Dr. Scott Donkin has explored the problems of poor sitting posture. Poor sitting posture may produce many of the same fatigability problems as poor standing posture or poor body mechanics. His work with corporations has confirmed what many doctors have observed for decades: poor sitting posture can lead to fatigue. Donkin states, "Fatigue is a common complaint among workers. It is often difficult to measure, but is frequently described as a vague tiredness or feeling of low energy, lack of enthusiasm, or weakness. The major causes [of fatigue among workers] include ... poor posture, chair support, as well as not properly fitting into your work station." Donkin has also highlighted the problems of poor sleeping posture, which may also contribute to fatigue.[2]

How common are these postural and biomechanical problems? Dr. Joseph Sweere is the chairman of the Department of Occupational Health at Northwestern College of Chiropractic and is the chairman of the Rehabilitation Review Panel for the Minnesota Department of Labor and Industry. He lectures throughout the world on the impact of biomechanics, posture, and ergonomics on health and safety. He recently reported on a study of 450 people in which he assessed the biomechanical stress index (BSI). Within this index he evaluated the various factors that caused a shift from an ideal center of gravity—forward, backward, right, or left.[3] Dr. Sweere found that roughly 33 percent of all the people tested had a deviation of the total body posture to the right or left of center. Roughly 27 percent had a deviation of the total body posture either forward or backward. He also found that those individuals were more likely to suffer fatigued muscles, which were more likely to result in injury.

In our discussion, Dr. Sweere theorized that such shifts in the center of gravity may be an important contributor to chronic fatigue, poor energy, and low vitality in a significant number of people. He suggested that this aspect of the fatigue connection is overlooked by most in the medical field.

There are three primary ways that body mechanics can be altered and lead to chronic fatigue and low vitality.

1. *Poor posture.* Many people become used to standing and walking with their shoulders slouched, rounded forward, their head hanging downward, their belly sagging forward, and their pelvis tipped

forward. Their sitting is no better, with legs crossed, shoulders forward, and back rounded. This effect of posture is mainly a behavioral issue related to habit and training. It can be unlearned and merely requires using proper technique when you sit, stand, and walk.

2. *Functional body mechanics.* There are several types of functional mechanical changes.

- *Changes in the spinal column.* Subluxation is a term used to describe a malposition of one bone with respect to the adjacent bone. This commonly occurs in the spine where one vertebra may tip sideways, rotate, or shift to the right or left. When such a shift occurs, all of the vertebrae above must compensate for the change. In many cases this can cause the head to shift off the midline, changing the center of gravity. This can lead to fatigability of the involved supportive muscles. If your posture or spinal mechanics are poor, it can restrict the movement of the rib cage and thus reduce the efficiency with which you breathe. Anything that reduces your breathing efficiency can also reduce your energy.

- *Changes in the muscles that hold up the skeleton.* When supportive muscles become weak or spastic, it changes the mechanical relationships of the spine. A classic example so common in the modern world is weak abdominal muscles. When your abdominal muscles become weakened and your belly begins to protrude forward, you experience a measurable shift in your spinal mechanics and movement of the center of gravity. Your body then recruits other supportive muscles to do the work of the abdominals and tries to correct the developing postural change. This is an inefficient process that requires extra energy to maintain.

- *Changes in the feet, knees, and hips.* Changes in these areas, which represent the foundation on which spinal mechanics are built, can cause the whole spinal column and its supporting muscles to compensate.

3. *Pathology and skeletal defects.* Significant postural changes can occur when there is a defect or deformity in the feet, knees, pelvis, or spine. One example is a fracture that has not healed in proper

alignment. A common condition known as spondylolisthesis, in which the bony arch of the 5th lumbar vertebra has fractured, separated, or weakened, often causes the body's center of gravity to shift forward. Another situation occurs in people who have one leg that is slightly shorter than the other. This can occur as a result of a fracture to one of the legs that may have caused it to lag behind in growth or simply as a common developmental defect. A short leg will cause the entire spine to shift laterally in compensation.

A common response given by people who have received treatment from chiropractic physicians is that they feel like they have more energy, more vitality. When you look at the impact of posture on energy and vitality, and realize that the adjustive, muscular, and postural techniques used by chiropractic physicians are designed to correct faulty body mechanics, it seems perfectly logical. Structure alters function. When body mechanics are structurally unsound, there is an enormous adverse effect on function. Many body functions can be impacted by problems of body mechanics. The one we're concerned with here happens to be the energy/fatigue connection.

Dr. Edward Farinelli, of Fort Collins, Colorado, conducted a case study of seventy patients with chronic fatigue to see how adjustment of the spine might affect fatigue symptoms. In the group receiving diversified adjustments of the spine, there was improvement in fatigue symptoms. However, relief was temporary. After several months, this group began receiving specific adjustments to the first and second cervical vertebrae (C1 and C2). All reported improvement that remained for over six months. Another group received specific adjustment of the C1-C2 area of the spine from the outset. In this group, ten out of ten patients reported long-term relief from their chronic fatigue symptoms.[4]

Farinelli does not provide many details about how his study was designed and carried out, so it is difficult to know how precisely his findings can be interpreted. However, results similar to his have been observed by other chiropractic physicians in private practice.

How might adjustment of the spine improve the symptoms of fatigue? The answer is not clear, and it would be inappropriate to attempt a detailed explanation in the context of a book as brief as this. However, the current evidence seems to point to an effect of adjustment of the spine on the nervous system and immune system. An article published in the *Journal of Manipulative and Physiological Therapeutics* described the chemical messengers that allow for communication between the nervous and immune systems. It was suggested that fixation of the spine (impaired movement between the two or more vertebrae) of the spine could have an adverse effect on the sympathetic nervous system and that this may in turn affect immune function.[5]

There are preliminary reports that suggest adjustment of the spine can have a beneficial effect on certain aspects of the immune response, specifically, the respiratory burst of white blood cells.[6] These studies were carried out after adjustment of the thoracic and lumbar areas of the spine (middle and low back). A direct effect of adjustment on the brain stem or autonomic nervous system may possibly have an effect on energy production. Research will likely uncover more over the years about the problems of poor body mechanics and the benefits of spinal adjustment on health.

Laboratory Tests

Assessment of posture and biomechanics is actually quite straightforward. Postural assessment is done using a plumb line postural analyzer, much like that used in engineering and building construction. These are either visual-based or computer-based. The plumb line system will be able to show whether your body has deviated forward, backward, or to one side. There are also clinics that utilize special pressure-sensitive foot plates to determine where the weight of the body is concentrated. This gives an indication of how the center of gravity has shifted.

Another method used is analysis of standing x-rays. Most other medical x-rays are taken with the patient lying down. This type of film provides useful information about disease and pathology, but not about spinal mechanics. Standing x-rays more accurately reflect how your body behaves under the demands of weight-bearing activity. They more accurately reflect the effect of gravity on body mechanics. Standing x-rays can be analyzed using precise measurements and mathematical formulas. The geometry of various spinal angles and curvatures has been well-studied. If your measurements deviate from the norm, corrective measures can be taken that are tailored to your specific situation.

Assessment of whether vertebral subluxations exist is usually done by manual palpation of the spinal column while sitting, lying, and moving.

Treatment

Treatment of fatigue that is due to imbalanced body mechanics often includes the following:

1. *Postural training.* Learn to walk, sit, lift, and sleep with posture that optimizes your body and muscle function. This can be done without the help of a health professional. However, most people have been engaged in poor posture for so long they do not know what optimum posture looks or feels like.

2. *Manipulation or adjustment of the spine, pelvis, knees, or feet.* Manipulation/adjustment can help restore normal function to the mechanics of the body by improving mobility, improving mechanics, restoring muscle tone and balance, and improving nervous system function.

3. *Muscle strengthening exercises.* If posture has been poor for years, a variety of muscle groups have likely become weak in order for the shift to occur. These muscles must be strengthened with specific exercises.

4. *Stretching.* When poor posture exists, there are always muscles that have become shortened and in many cases hypertonic (excessively contracted). Stretching that focuses on these groups is vital. General stretching is essential to move the center of gravity back to normal.

5. *Orthotics.* Many postural problems originate in the feet. The Leaning Tower of Pisa leans because the foundation has

sunk into the ground. Likewise, if your feet (or foot) are not functioning properly, they provide an unstable foundation and all structures above them change as a result. Orthotics are inserts placed into the shoes used to correct spinal and foot mechanics.

6. *Massage.* Massage is invaluable in restoring muscle balance, tone, and flexibility.

7. *Nutritional support.* All metabolic processes of muscle require nutrients to function at their peak. Likewise, all connective tissue requires nutrients to maintain integrity and strength. Remember, one of the first tissues to suffer in vitamin C deficiency is connective tissue—the stuff that holds you together. There are many other nutrients essential to this process.

Manipulation of the spine and extremities has been practiced for centuries. Modern chiropractic will celebrate its 100th anniversary in 1995, the profession having grown to more than 50,000 doctors nationwide. This also reflects a growing interest in manipulation among other health professionals. In the March 1994 issue of *Family Practice News,* it was noted that in the next twenty-five years, "physicians who do not know how to do manipulation will be at a disadvantage." The American Academy of Family Physicians recently voted to recognize manipulation for continuing medical education credit.[7] Chiropractic and osteopathy are presently the primary professions licensed to perform manipulation in the United States.

In Review

1. A large percentage of the body's energy production is directed toward holding the body in space.

2. Poor posture or altered body mechanics can lead to chronic fatigue and low vitality in some people.

3. Static loading caused by poor body mechanics can lead to increased lactic acid buildup in the muscles, decreased

oxygen delivery to the tissues, and decreased elimination of toxins and waste products.

4. The body expends the least amount of energy when balanced properly over its center of gravity.

5. The body expends the most amount of energy whenever it deviates from its center of gravity.

6. Chiropractic care and postural training techniques can often improve energy immensely.

ght sweats, chronic fatigue, memory impairment, and sore throat.[9] According to a report by the National Research Council, 87 different chemicals have been associated with fatigue, 179 with weakness, with pain, and 64 with pain disorders.[10]

The nose is the only part of the brain that is directly exposed to the outside world. According to Iris Bell, M.D., Ph.D., odors (from toxic chemicals) inhaled through the nose have easier access to the brain and can disrupt emotions, memory, sleep, immunity, and energy by interfering with the limbic system.[11]

Altered Neurotransmitters. Neurotransmitters are chemical messengers that carry information throughout the brain and body. Serotonin is a neurotransmitter found to be low in FMS. Serotonin is made in the brain from the dietary amino acid tryptophan. Tryptophan has also been found to be low in FMS. In one study, 75 percent of people with FMS produced antibodies against their own serotonin in the brain.[12] One family of drugs, called SSRI, or selective serotonin reuptake inhibitors, have provided relief for some FMS patients. Included are Prozac and Zoloft. However, these drugs still do not address the underlying factors that alter brain metabolism.

Aluminum Toxicity. Aluminum blocks the ATP molecule, the primary energy molecule in the body. Malic acid and magnesium are among the most powerful aluminum detoxifiers known.[13;14] Both nutrients have been found in controlled studies to relieve the pain of FMS.

Stress. Paul Davidson, M.D., internist and author of *Chronic Muscle Pain Syndrome,* contends that fibromyalgia is the body's painful reaction to deep-rooted stress, the most common consequences being fatigue and exhaustion. Other symptoms that accompany this "stress reaction" may include migraine headaches, numbness and tingling in the extremities, temperature and humidity sensitivity, tension and poor stress tolerance, anxiety, depression, and general lack of well-being.[15] While stress may be a factor in FMS, there are far too many biochemical abnormalities being discovered to attribute the syndrome solely to stress.

Food Allergy or Intolerance. Muscle pain and fatigue are among the manifestations of food intolerance in some people. In 1993, a

Chapter 12

Chronic Muscle Pain:
The Pain and Fatigue of Fibromyalgia

IF YOUR MUSCLES ACHE all over, you are tired and fatigued, and you have difficulty sleeping, there is a good chance you suffer from a condition known as fibromyalgia syndrome (FMS). It is characterized by general muscle aches all over the body, with tenderness at very specific points on certain muscle groups. In the United States, an estimated three to six million people suffer from fibromyalgia, but this figure may be only the tip of the iceberg. Some rheumatologists and chiropractors believe that fibromyalgia is the most common condition seen in their practices, especially in women between the ages of 20 and 50.

Fibromyalgia is characterized by widespread pain and tenderness. Joints are not typically involved, which makes this different from arthritis. Generally, the symptoms are located in muscles of the hips, back, shoulder, and neck. Chronic pain is accompanied by stiffness, especially in the morning and late evening, that is also more prominent in the neck, spine, shoulders, and hips. Most people with fibromyalgia have had their pain for months to years. Symptoms usually arise gradually and subtly, often following a sprain, strain, whiplash, or other trauma. Some report the onset of symptoms following viral, bacterial, or parasitic infection. Indeed, many patients in describing their symptoms say it feels like they have the flu, with its accompanying achiness of muscles and joints. The hallmark of fibromyalgia is the existence of multiple tender points located in well-defined areas. However, people with this disorder are often unaware that the pain is so localized and feel as though it exists all over.

Fatigue is one of the most significant complaints of those with fibromyalgia, affecting up to 90 percent of such individuals.[1] Indeed, many studies now suggest that chronic fatigue syndrome and fibromyalgia syndrome are the same disorder. Fibromyalgia is more common in those who are not physically fit. Those who exercise regularly are not as likely to develop the condition.

One of the most common characteristics of FMS is the patterns of disrupted sleep. Those with FMS seem to fall asleep without much difficulty, but they wake frequently during the night, especially during normal deep sleep cycles. This may in part account for their fatigue and waking without feeling rested (though it is believed that additional factors are involved). Magnesium deficiency, which appears to be somewhat common among those with FMS, is also common among those with sleep difficulties.

Shortness of breath is one of the common characteristics of FMS, affecting an estimated 84 percent. FMS is characterized by significant changes in brain chemistry. One such change involves the neurochemical serotonin and the amino acid tryptophan. Jay Goldstein, M.D., author of *Chronic Fatigue Syndromes: The Limbic Hypothesis*, believes that FMS/CFS is related to disordered function of the part of the brain known as the limbic system, which is highly interconnected with the immune system, endocrine system, and emotions. Painful jaws, or TMJ (temporomandibular joint) dysfunction, is another symptom somewhat common in FMS. People with FMS/CFS are often highly sensitive to chemicals, odors, noises, bright lights, touch, and other forms of stimulation.[2]

Fibromyalgia can occur in the presence or absence of other conditions. It is known to occur in association with rheumatoid arthritis, osteoarthritis, and hypothyroidism.[3,4] No single cause has been found for fibromyalgia, and the causes may vary from person to person. The following factors are among those associated with

fibromyalgia. As you read this, recognize that fibro[   ] understood condition. New studies are being publi[   ] that will add to or modify the discussion presente[   ]

Viral Infection. Many patients report the onset [   ] toms and fatigue associated with a cold, the flu, m[   ] some other viral infection. A viral infection may cau[   ] of the immune response, sending it into a hypervigil[   ] prolonged hyperactive state it secretes a family of ch[   ] as cytokines. High levels of cytokines have been fou[   ] with FMS/CFS and may be responsible for many of t[   ]

Intestinal Parasite Infection. Dr. Leo Galland repor[   ] of 218 patients with complaints of chronic fatigue, mus[   ] cle weakness, and intestinal symptoms. Sixty-one [   ] infected with the parasite *Giardia lamblia*. Thirteen [   ] enced a complete cure after giardia treatment, 21 experie[   ] improvement, eight had some benefit, and six had no i[   ] Treatment included grapefruit seed extract, the herb *Arte*[   ] a combination of the above, the drug quinacrine, or the d[   ] idazole for ten days.[6]

Lyme Disease. One manifestation of Lyme disease, caus[   ] tion of the bacteria *Borrelia burgdorferi*, is fibromyalgia a[   ] fatigue. According to an article in the *Journal of the Ame*[   ] *ical Association*, fibromyalgia that is triggered by Lyme d[   ] not respond well to antibiotic therapy.[7] A study was publi[   ] *Annals of Internal Medicine* that looked at the effectiveness [   ] otic treatment in patients with chronic fatigue, fibromyal[   ] positive Lyme disease blood test, but *who did not have* [   ] *symptoms of Lyme disease.* The researchers concluded that [   ] such patients the risks of antibiotics in this situation exce[   ] benefits, though two to four weeks of oral antibiotics appea[   ] quate to eliminate the infectious agent.[8] (See chapter 13.)

Chemical Exposure. A common complaint of patients wit[   ] sure to chemicals or chemical toxicity is fatigue, headaches, ar[   ] cle pain. According to Gunnar Heuser, M.D., Ph.D., of the Un[   ] of California at Los Angeles, toxic chemical exposure often c[   ] flu-like syndrome which includes headaches, muscle aches and[   ] study was reported on patients with rheumatoid arthritis who consumed a vegetarian diet for three weeks. Seventy percent of this group reported improved symptoms.[16] While FMS is fundamentally different than rheumatoid arthritis, some doctors have begun to look at the role of diet in FMS as well. Dr. Russell Jaffe, director of Serammune Physician's Laboratory, reported on their pilot study of FMS patients who were tested for delayed reactions to foods and chemicals. When offending foods and chemicals were identified and removed from the patient's environment, coupled with measures designed to enhance immune function, patient improvement was greater than 85 percent.[17]

Altered Intestinal Permeability. Altered intestinal permeability is being associated with a growing number of muscle and skeletal problems. A preliminary study conducted at the Cheney Clinic in collaboration with Great Smokies Diagnostic Laboratory suggests that most people with chronic fatigue *syndrome* may have increased intestinal permeability.[18]

Essential Fatty Acids. In a study of 63 patients with post-viral fatigue, muscle pain, and psychiatric symptoms, EFA supplementation caused improvement in 74 percent of patients after one month and 85 percent after three months (23 and 17 percent respectively for placebo group). Dosages included 36 mg GLA, 17 mg EPA, 11 mg DHA, 255 mg LA.[19]

Thyroid Problems. Hypothyroidism is an endocrine disorder that should be ruled out with blood tests. It can cause symptoms of FMS.

Accidents or Trauma. Twenty to fifty percent of the cases of fibromyalgia follow a specific injury or trauma.[20] Whiplash injuries of the neck are known to lead to FMS in some people. This may be due to injury of the soft tissue of the spine (muscles, ligaments, tendons, connective tissue) that can occur with whiplash. This may, in turn, alter thyroid function.

Biochemical. Researchers are beginning to uncover blocks or defects in the body's biochemical machinery. This may be one of the most promising areas of research. Some have found deficiency of malic acid and magnesium to be a problem. Supplementation with these nutrients has reduced muscle soreness and fatigue. An article published in the *Journal of Nutritional Medicine* reviewed a study of people with fibromyalgia who took 300 to 600 mg of magnesium per day and 1,200 to 2,400 mg of malic acid per day for four to eight weeks. All patients reported significant relief of pain within 48 hours of treatment and had a measurable improvement in the severity of their muscle tender points.[21] Malic acid is a normal part of the citric acid cycle that is vital to energy production. Since this study, many doctors have reported success in treating a subset of FMS patients with malic acid and magnesium. In my opinion, it still solves only a small portion of the FMS puzzle.

Researchers writing in the *Journal of Advancement in Medicine* have also found that people with fibromyalgia have impaired thiamin (B_1) status and that they may benefit significantly by taking a special form of vitamin B_1 known as thiamin pyrophosphate (TPP). The scientists compared the response of people with different types of chronic pain syndromes including those with FMS, and measured their response to TPP. Those with FMS improved markedly on TPP, while those with other pain syndromes did not. This caused the researchers to conclude, "The pain experienced by patients with fibromyalgia is related to a biochemical lesion and this condition has a uniquely different cause which requires appropriate nutrient therapy rather than the traditional approach with analgesics [pain relievers]."[22] Another study by the same researcher showed that there are significant alterations in energy metabolism in fibromyalgia, namely decreased ATP.[23] These studies may explain, in part, why patients with FMS do not experience much relief from pain relievers such as aspirin or ibuprofen.

Despite some promising findings, fibromyalgia remains a painful and poorly understood condition. There appear to be no universal causes and no single treatment that is effective for every person.

Signs and Symptoms

Fatigue	Tenderness at 11 of 18 specific
Chronic aching	muscle points
Sleep disturbance	Stiffness (especially morning)
Anxiety	Pain

Intestinal complaints   Depression (possible)
Shortness of breath

Laboratory Tests

There are no laboratory tests that can confirm a diagnosis of fibromyalgia. This diagnosis is made by finding tenderness on at least 11 of 18 specific points on the body musculature. Standard laboratory findings are usually not revealing unless another accompanying disease condition exists.[24,25]

Some doctors who practice functional medicine or holistic medicine may order certain functional tests in an effort to determine if a metabolic imbalance is contributing to the muscle pain and fatigue. Some of the tests include:

• Organic acid analysis

• Amino acid analysis

• Heavy metal analysis

• Intestinal permeability test

• Vitamin and mineral tests

• Comprehensive parasitology

• IgG tests for food hypersensitivity

• ELISA/ACT for delayed reaction to foods and chemicals

Treatment

There are no generally effective medical treatments for fibromyalgia. Medications commonly used include aspirin, ibuprofen, indomethacin, and others. However, while effective in relieving the aches and pains of injuries and other musculoskeletal pain, these drugs have been compared and found to be no more effective than placebos in treating FMS.[26] Another drug, the tricyclic antidepressant amitriptyline (Elavil), is helpful for some patients with FMS but is by no means a panacea. It does have immediate side effects in some people including dry mouth, confusion, weakness, irregular heartbeat, seizure, and alopecia (hair loss).[27] The long-term side effects are unclear, though the drug is not believed to be addictive.

Nutritional support has been helpful in many patients. As noted above, recent research has begun to point to certain metabolic pathways as a focal point of some of the fibromyalgia symptoms. For this reason, nutrients that correct this metabolic imbalance are being used by some doctors. Nutrients most commonly used include: magnesium, vitamins B_1, B_2, B_6, and C, malic acid, and manganese. In one study, administration of 5-hydroxy tryptophan (a form of tryptophan) improved all clinical symptoms in patients with FMS.[28]

Electroacupuncture has been used with some success. In one study, FMS patients were treated using electroacupuncture at four common points over a three-week period. Those receiving the treatments experienced greater improvement in symptoms including pain, sleep quality, and pain threshold.[29] In a study published in the *British Medical Journal,* patients given homeopathic *Rhus toxicodendron* for FMS did better in all categories than those on placebo.[30]

Detoxification can be helpful. One underlying feature common to many cases of fibromyalgia is cellular toxicity or disordered metabolism. This may be true whether due to chemical exposure, allergies, thyroid problems, viral infection, parasitic infection, nutrient deficiency, aluminum, mercury, or lead toxicity, or altered intestinal permeability. By using a detoxification program, such as that developed by Jeffrey Bland, Ph.D., one can begin to restore balance in many seemingly unrelated situations. For instance, Dr. Bland found that patients placed on a detoxification program experienced an increase in the amount of magnesium that entered the cell (which is desirable) even though magnesium was not given.

Some people with fibromyalgia benefit from exercise. A study reported in the *American Journal of Medicine* showed that when aerobic conditioning was undertaken, the symptoms of fibromyalgia improved. The authors reported, "... cardiovascular fitness training is feasible in patients with fibrositis/fibromyalgia and such training improves subjective measurements of pain-reporting behavior."[31] If you desire to begin an exercise program, do so under the guidance of a doctor, begin gradually, and make sure the exercise is tailored to your existing level of fitness.

Stress management is vitally important if you wish to recover from fibromyalgia. A stretching routine that incorporates deep breathing is also important. Some patients find meditation extremely helpful. Yoga is one good technique that incorporates both stretching, deep breathing, and if you choose, meditation.

The jury is still out on effective treatment of FMS. The future will likely hold many promising therapies. Keep in mind that the best therapy will likely be one that integrates nutrition, diet therapy, mind/body work, medication in some cases, exercise, lifestyle modification, and other modalities. A supportive team approach, with different professionals working together, may be best.

In Review

1. Fibromyalgia is a condition of chronic muscle pain accompanied by exhaustion and fatigue.

2. There is no single cause of fibromyalgia.

3. It seems to strike women between the ages of 20 and 50. About 25 percent of those with FMS are men.

4. FMS sometimes follows trauma such as an auto accident, but may be related to viral infection, parasite infection, chemical exposure, or other factors.

5. FMS does not respond well to drug treatment.

6. There is encouraging evidence that FMS is, in part, due to disrupted metabolism and that specific nutritional supplementation may have promise.

7. Stress management is an important factor in recovering from FMS.

8. Recovery from FMS requires an integrated approach that may include diet and nutritional therapy, stress management, exercise, stretching, meditation, analgesics, therapy, and detoxification.

Chapter 13

Infections That May Cause Fatigue

CHRONIC INFECTIONS BY bacteria, viruses, parasites, or yeast can result in fatigue. Some of these infections can go unrecognized for months or years. It may take some detective work on the part of you and your doctor to determine whether your fatigue might be due to a chronic infection. In many cases, laboratory tests are available that can help identify the organism that is causing problems.

The greatest hint that you may suffer from a hidden infection is if your fatigue came on gradually or abruptly after a bacterial, viral, parasitic, or fungal infection. In some cases, it is not easy to make this association. Nonetheless, it is important that you retrace your steps and identify the time your fatigue began.

If your doctor suspects an infectious agent as a part of your problem, don't be too quick to jump at the prospect of antibiotic therapy. Remember, antibiotics do not kill viruses, so they would be of little use in a viral infection. Antibiotics do not kill yeast or fungi. In fact, they may aggravate a yeast or fungal infection. Antibiotics do kill bacteria. However, the problem of antibiotic-resistant bacteria has become epidemic. Antibiotics can no longer be used with impunity. If your doctor recommends antibiotics for suspected infection you may wish to ask the following questions:

1. Has a culture shown this to be a bacterial infection?
2. Do you know the type of bacteria involved?

3. Have you determined to which antibiotic the bacteria is sensitive? Have you performed a sensitivity test?

4. What is the resistance pattern of this bacterium in this region of the country?

5. What is the minimum amount of time that I must take the antibiotic in order for it to be effective?

6. Can we use an antibiotic with a narrow spectrum of action and still get the job done?

7. What are the expected side effects of taking this antibiotic?

8. What other things might I do to optimize my immune response?

Many doctors and researchers believe that in order for one to become seriously ill as a result of invasion by microorganisms, their resistance must in some way be compromised. Physician and researcher Thomas McKeown summarized this idea when he said, "...the conclusion which seems inescapable is that the influences which determine man's response to infectious disease—genetics, nutritional, environmental, behavioral, as well as medical—are infinitely complex, and we need to be very cautious before assuming that we fully understand the infection, or that we have in our hands the certain means of their control."[1]

I have previously presented an extensive discussion of the dietary, nutritional, lifestyle, environmental, and psychological factors that influence our resistance to infections *(Beyond Antibiotics)*. It has become clear to me that much more is required to succumb to bacteria and viruses than simple exposure to them. Furthermore, in order to fully recover (especially if the infection is chronic) one must make positive changes in the areas known to enhance immunity.

Some of the more common hidden infections associated with fatigue are listed below.

Infectious Mononucleosis. Infectious mononucleosis commonly affects adolescents and college students, but can affect anyone from adolescence to adulthood. The symptoms include swollen glands, extreme fatigue and tiredness, and sore throat. The fatigue of mononucleosis usually lasts for several weeks, but can persist for months or years. If it persists for many months or years it is often referred to as post-viral fatigue syndrome (PVFS). These infections are caused by the Epstein-Barr virus. Other viruses can contribute to PVFS as well.

One reason fatigue may persist is that virus infection can seriously undermine nutritional status, which then impairs immune function. Nutritional supplementation can be enormously helpful to those with post-viral fatigue. Two important studies illustrate this point.

During 1988 and 1989, Dr. Allen Stewart studied the blood nutrient levels of 16 patients with post-viral fatigue syndrome. He found that 14 of the 16 patients had at least one abnormal nutrient result. For example, B1 and B6 levels were low in more than half of those in whom it was measured. Zinc was low in 8 of 16 patients. Magnesium was low in 9 of 15 people. Each of the patients was given a vitamin and mineral supplement that addressed their deficiencies. Of the 16 receiving supplements, eight subjects had either full or good improvement.[2] Stewart's findings are significant, but there are other nutrients important in recovery from PVFS.

In 1990, researchers from Scotland and Canada reported on their study of essential fatty acid supplementation in 63 patients with post-viral fatigue, exhaustion, weakness, poor concentration, and other symptoms common to PVFS. In the fatigued patients, red cell levels of omega-3 and omega-6 fatty acids were well below normal. Each was then given a supplement containing 80 percent evening primrose oil (a rich source of gamma-linolenic acid [GLA]) and 20 percent concentrated fish oil (a rich source of eicosapentaenoic acid [EPA] and docosahexaenoic acid [DHA]). EFA supplementation caused improvement in 74 percent of patients after one month and 85 percent after three months (23 and 17 percent respectively for placebo group). Not only did symptoms improve, but red cell fatty acid levels returned to normal.[3]

My wife developed post-viral fatigue syndrome several years ago. It was during a period of high stress at work coupled with numerous responsibilities in church and community activities. She became worn out and came down with acute mononucleosis. She was exhausted, sleepy, and spent most of her hours in bed or on the couch resting. We used a variety of methods including nutrition and botanical medicine to improve her stamina and energy, but her fatigue lasted for nearly one year after the initial infection. The main reason I believe the symptoms persisted for so long is that she returned to work far too early. This should be a lesson to all of us. Rest is one of the most important ingredients to recovery. If we push ourselves too far, even the healthiest people can become ill. Don't underestimate the demands that work and civic obligations take on your body and mind.

Yeast Infection. Infection by the yeast *Candida albicans* contributes to a condition called candida-related complex (CRC). William Crook, M.D., author of *Chronic Fatigue Syndrome and the Yeast Connection,* has reported that fatigue is a common manifestation of people with this infection.[4] *Candida albicans* is a normal inhabitant of the human intestinal tract that generally lives in harmony with the hundreds of other species of microbes with which they reside. When antibiotics are used extensively, beneficial bacteria that live in the gut are killed off and the yeast may grow uncontrolled. This leads to excessive levels of *Candida albicans* in the gut, which can lead to food intolerance, intestinal upset, immune deficiency, headaches, skin disorders, fatigue, and a variety of other symptoms.

In 1989 and 1990, Carol Jessop, M.D., Assistant Clinical Professor at the University of California at San Francisco, presented case studies of more than 1,000 patients with chronic fatigue. She reported that 88 percent of these patients had a history of *recurrent antibiotic treatment* (as a child, adolescent, or adult).[5] Leo Galland, M.D., was the keynote speaker at a 1988 conference on candida-related complex. In his address, he noted that antibiotics were a precipitating factor in 82 percent of patients with CRC.[6]

The major symptoms of candida-related complex (CRC) include:

Fatigue or lethargy	Bloating, intestinal gas
Poor memory	Vaginal itching, burning,
Feeling "spacy" or "unreal"	discharge

Numbness, burning, tingling	Prostatitis
Insomnia	Premenstrual tension, PMS
Muscle aches, weakness	Attacks of anxiety or crying
Abdominal pain	Shaking or irritability when
Constipation	hungry

Other symptoms include:

Headaches, sinusitis	Food sensitivity or intolerance
Moodiness	Mucus in stools
White tongue	Rectal itching
Tendency to bruise easily	Hoarseness, loss of voice
Chronic rashes, itching	Nasal itching

Lyme Disease. Lyme disease is caused by a spiral-shaped bacterium called *Borrelia burgdorferi*. It is contracted from the bite of an infected deer tick. While the tick is attached it injects the bacteria into the human bloodstream, where it begins to do its dirty work. The first sign to appear after being bitten by the tick is the appearance of a rash called erythema migrans. The rash usually begins two to thirty-two days after a tick bite or known tick exposure. The rash is unusual in that it commonly begins as a small circle. The outer ring of the circle continues to expand and retains a red outer border—almost like a bull's eye. Not all bites appear this way, however. Some patients experience multiple skin lesions. Other symptoms may include muscle aches, dizziness, heart palpitations, headaches, arthritis or joint swelling, fibromyalgia, and symptoms that may mimic many other conditions. Some patients describe feeling like they have the flu. Some people diagnosed with multiple sclerosis have actually later been found to have Lyme disease.

The standard treatment for confirmed Lyme disease is a 10-day to 30-day course of oral doxycycline, amoxicillin, or amoxicillin plus probenecid for early infections. Many infections require a combination of intravenous antibiotics for some months followed by oral antibiotics. Antibiotic therapy can be helpful in alleviating the symptoms of Lyme disease. However, many doctors believe that Lyme disease is overdiagnosed and overtreated, and that substantial numbers of people are receiving antibiotics for a disease that they do not have. This leads to antibiotic overuse and all the problems that can follow. According to an article in the *Journal of the American Medical Association,* of 788 patients referred for suspected Lyme disease, 57 percent were found not to have the disease.[7]

This report by Dr. Allen C. Steere has received widespread criticism because of problems with methodology and various assumptions made by his group. Some of the criticism has been voiced by Lyme disease patients and by other researchers. For example, some researchers charge that Steere used his own test as a control when this test has never been shown to be more accurate than other available tests. Many feel that the greatest impediment to diagnosis is the failure of doctors to acknowledge, recognize, and properly treat the infection. The critics of Dr. Steere believe the disease has serious medical ramifications and that his article has continued to fuel the skepticism of the medical community.[8]

If you receive a positive test for Lyme disease you should probably have it repeated just to be sure. There can be false positives with these tests, and you would not want to undergo antibiotic therapy needlessly. If the test is positive, you may benefit from antibiotic therapy, especially if the infection is caught in its early stage. In addition, supportive measures should be used to build immunity.

A new test for Lyme disease looks very promising. It is based on a technique used in genetic research called a polymerase chain reaction (PCR). This test uses a sample taken from joint fluid which is assayed for the presence of bacterial genetic material. In a report in the *New England Journal of Medicine* the test was found to detect *B. burgdorferi* in 85 percent of patients with Lyme arthritis and none of the control patients (without Lyme disease).[9] This test may more accurately identify who is a candidate for antibiotic therapy and who is not.

If you suspect you may have Lyme disease, it is vital that you find a doctor knowledgeable in this area, since not all doctors are familiar with the complexities of this diagnosis. Highlighting this is a figure from Dr. Joseph McDade of the CDC that in Connecticut, 82 percent of the cases of Lyme disease are reported by 7 percent of the doctors. Appropriate treatment is critical to halt the progression of this infection.

Hepatitis. Hepatitis is an inflammation of the liver that is often caused by a virus (but may be caused by other agents, such as alcohol). People who develop hepatitis often suffer from extreme fatigue and lethargy. While jaundice and enlarged liver are common findings, they are not always present. A blood test can determine whether you suffer from hepatitis.

Other Infections. Many different organisms can cause low-grade infections that lead to fatigue. Further, an infection may be localized to one or more different body systems. For example, vaginal infection by Candida, trichomonas, or chlamydia can lead to fatigue. Likewise, sinus infection by *Streptococcus pneumoniae* can lead to chronic stuffiness that leads to fatigue. In fact, proper treatment of sinusitis can often remedy the symptoms of fatigue. Chronic pelvic infection can lead to fatigue in women. Chronic intestinal infection can also lead to fatigue.

Other infections that can contribute to chronic fatigue include:

Cytomegalovirus	Toxoplasmosis
Tuberculosis	AIDS (HIV)
Syphilis	Human Herpes virus 6
Coxsackie virus	Herpes simplex I and II
Protozoans	

Many people with fatigue, especially chronic fatigue syndrome, have become obsessed with finding a single cause. They seek out physician after physician, and understandably so, in hopes that one will identify the culprit. With regard to hidden infections, I would resist the temptation to hang all my hopes on the diagnosis. There is some sound reasoning behind this advice. Suppose you've traveled from clinic to clinic and finally found a doctor who did the serological test showing you have high antibody titers to Epstein-Barr virus. Now what do you do? There is no specific medical treatment for EBV infection, so you are left with a diagnosis without a cure. If a bacterial infection is discovered and an appropriate antibiotic is available, great. That may be the first step on your road to recovery.

Just remember, infections can disrupt numerous body systems that must also be healed. Eliminating the microorganism is, in my opinion, only the initial phase of the treatment—not the whole treatment.

A sensible approach to these disorders is to assume that if an infection has taken place (and perhaps exists presently), it may have disrupted your metabolism, immune function, digestion, nutritional status, endocrine function, and other body processes. The task at hand then becomes "How do we optimize function in multiple body systems?" In the case of Dr. Tom, which I'll share later, he was found to have high antibody titers to EBV and *Borrelia burgdorferi.* This gave him an initial sense of relief: "Now I know what I have." But this was followed shortly by, "What do I do about it?" I'll describe the assessment and treatment approach in chapter 27.

Laboratory Tests

Most doctors will probably order a CBC with a differential blood count to begin. The differential count is helpful because the ratio of white blood cells called neutrophils, lymphocytes, and monocytes gives some indication of whether a viral or bacterial infection might be present. An ESR, or sed rate, may also be performed. Beyond this, many of the tests administered are specific to the disorder suspected. For example, if hepatitis is suspected you must test for the antibodies or antigen specific to the hepatitis virus. If Epstein-Barr virus infection is suspected, antibodies to this virus may be tested for.

Most tests involve taking a sample of the area of concern (blood, lung secretions, vaginal secretions, urine, etc.) and either culturing for the organism or testing for antibodies to the organism. A skin test may be done (as in tuberculosis) or an x-ray may be taken (as in pneumonia or sinusitis).

Intestinal Parasites

A growing number of doctors recognize intestinal parasites as a cause of fatigue in their patients. I've chosen to discuss parasitic infection separately for two reasons. First, many doctors in the United States do not give parasitic infection serious consideration because they believe it is uncommon (a thing of the past). Second, there have been recent advances in testing and diagnosis of which many doctors and patients are unaware. By one estimate, diarrheal disease caused by intestinal infection is the third leading cause of illness in the U.S.

Leo Galland, M.D., reported on a study of 218 patients whose main complaint was chronic fatigue. The parasite *Giardia lamblia* was identified in 61 patients. Cure of giardiasis resulted in clearing of fatigue in 70 percent of the patients treated. According to Dr. Galland, "This study shows that giardiasis can present with fatigue as the major manifestation, accompanied by minor gastrointestinal complaints and sometimes by myalgia and other symptoms suggestive of myalgic encephalomyelitis. It indicates that *G. lamblia* may be a common cause of CFS, at least in the United States."[10]

Intestinal parasites have been associated with increased intestinal permeability, food intolerance, malabsorption, autoimmune disease, skin conditions, psychological disorders such as depression, muscle and joint disease, as well as the more common gastrointestinal illness.[11]

Parasite infection can occur from drinking contaminated well or city water, from eating in a restaurant where food is prepared by a contaminated individual, from contact with your kids who attend day care, from travel to a foreign country, from backpacking in the mountains, or many other circumstances. I once counseled a woman who developed severe fatigue several weeks after returning from a trip to Latin America. It persisted for eight months before I saw her. During those eight months, none of her physicians considered nor tested for parasites. The stool analysis identified the parasite *Blastocystis hominis*. Other tests showed she had low secretory IgA (an important antibody defense in the gut) and malabsorption. Nancy did not improve until she completed a program to eliminate parasites.

I share this story because this is a common theme. It is possible your doctor has not considered parasites as a possible cause of your fatigue. Many doctors are only gradually becoming aware of the rising frequency with which parasitic infection occurs in the U.S.

The recent case of Milwaukee illustrates this point. In 1993, 400,000 people became infected by a one-celled organism called cryptosporidium. The infection was acquired through the city's water supply. Though this is an unusually large number of people, it suggests that parasitic infection is becoming more common than one might think.

Parasites can affect anyone. In those who test positive for parasites we often find one or more of the following in their history:

1. Backpacking or camping trip
2. Travel to a foreign country
3. Children in day care
4. Consumption of restaurant food prepared by infected food handler
5. No remarkable history. In some cases, there is no real incident or experience that would suggest exposure to parasites has occurred.

Signs and Symptoms

Symptoms associated with parasitic infection can be divided into four primary areas:

- Gastrointestinal: bloating, gas, heartburn, diarrhea, constipation, cramping, bleeding, etc.
- Neurobehavioral or psychological: depression, fatigue, anxiety, memory impairment, sluggishness, inability to concentrate
- Allergy: food intolerance or allergy, airborne allergy
- Immunological: infection susceptibility, autoimmune disease, poor immune repair

Laboratory Tests

Conventional stool screening tests used by most doctors often do not detect parasites when present. Recent advances in sampling, staining, and microscopy have improved the accuracy of parasite identification immensely. Your doctor should request two (or three) of the following types of stool samples in order to obtain the most accurate results:

- Rectal swab. A small sample of mucus is taken from the rectum by swabbing with a cotton-tipped applicator.
- Random formed stool. This sample is obtained by defecating into a container and taking a small sample of stool. This is the type of sample commonly used and does provide useful information when used with other tests. It is not as useful when it is the only sample analyzed.
- Purge stool. A laxative is consumed, which flushes (or purges) the contents of the bowels. This helps detect parasites that may cling tenaciously to the gut lining and be undetectable in the random formed stool.

According to Lee and Barrie at Great Smokies Diagnostic Laboratory, the identification of parasites was most accurate when a combination of the random stool and the purge was used.[12]

Treatment

The common parasites *Giardia lamblia, E. histolytica, Blastocystis hominis, Dientamoeba fragilis,* etc., are generally treated with one of a number of drugs, including metronidazole, quinacrine, and iodoquinol. Because of undesired side effects, drug-resistant parasites, and desire to use effective natural preparations, some doctors have begun to use botanicals with antiprotozoan activity. Included are: *Artemisia annua,* garlic, Hydrastis (goldenseal), grapefruit seed extract, black walnut bark, and others. Probiotics such as acidophilus, bifidus, and other normal gut inhabitants are also being used as part of a comprehensive parasite treatment.[13]

Treatment of intestinal parasites should include the following:

- Substances that eradicate the parasites. This may include drugs, nutrients, or botanicals.
- Avoidance of offending foods. Parasitic infection often contributes to food intolerance.
- Substances that restore gut ecology. This may include probiotics such as acidophilus or bifidus, and substance that enhance the growth of these organisms such as fructooligosaccharides.

- Elimination of the source of parasites. This means investigating family members, water supplies, day care, and other possible sources.
- Substances or lifestyle practices aimed at normalizing secretory IgA levels. This is an antibody that protects the gut from infection.
- Nutrients that are deficient. Parasitic infection often leads to poor absorption and nutrient deficiency.
- Substances that rebuild the gut lining. Leaky gut and inflammatory changes often occur with parasitic infection. Nutrients that rebuild the gut mucosa are discussed in chapter 2.

The Immune System

By now most people are aware that the immune system is what protects us from the millions of microbes and foreign substances with which we come in contact. Many patients with chronic fatigue have alterations in immune function that play a role in their illness.*

The white blood cells are the soldiers of the immune system. When your doctor orders a white count he or she is performing the most basic assessment of your immune system. The white count looks at the number, size, and shape of cells called neutrophils, lymphocytes, monocytes, basophils, and eosinophils. There are standard ratios of each of these that normally exist in a healthy person.

The part of the immune system we'll discuss focuses on the lymphocytes and consists of two primary components: the cellular and the humoral systems. The cellular component consists of T-lymphocytes, or T-cells, so named because of their maturation in the thymus gland, the walnut-sized gland behind your breastbone. There are four basic subcategories of T-cells. They include T-helper cells, T-suppressor cells, T-killer cells, and memory cells. The B-lympho-

---

*It is beyond the scope of this book to present a detailed discussion of the immune system. However, no discussion of chronic fatigue would be complete without at least a brief discussion of the immune system.

cytes, or B-cells, form the major component of the humoral immune system. The T- and B-cells communicate in a beautifully orchestrated manner that also involves the nervous system. A brief note about the above cells will give you a basic understanding of what the immune system does.

T-helper cells. T-helper cells are warned of a threat by other cells. Their job is to alert and arouse other components of the immune system. Some people who are fatigued and many people with chronic fatigue *syndrome* have inadequate numbers of T-helpers, so they do not mount a potent immune response to invaders. Such people would be more susceptible to infection by viruses, bacteria, and parasites.

T-suppressor cells. These cells announce to other immune cells that the threat is over. Their signals cause a suppression of the immune response. Some people with chronic fatigue have too many T-suppressor cells, and the immune system is in an overall state of sluggishness or suppression.

The ratio of T-helpers to suppressors in healthy people is about 1.8:1, meaning there are almost twice as many helpers as suppressors. With this ratio, the immune system runs most efficiently. Many people with chronic illness have a ratio of helpers to suppressors that is too high or too low. The result can be infection susceptibility or an immune system that is too vigilant and attacks other body tissues.

T-killer cells. These cells actually carry out the business of killing the invaders. They engage in a form of hand-to-hand combat by bumping into the invader and injecting a powerful substance to kill it.

T-memory cells. Memory cells keep a record of past encounters so that if the same invader returns, a rapid immune response to it can be mounted.

B-cells. These cells are part of the circulating immune system. They manufacture antibodies, a specialized class of proteins made to recognize and bind to foreign substances. The antibodies are manufactured against the invader, released into the bloodstream, and attach to the surface of the invader (forming an immune complex).

This neutralizes the invader until the cleanup crew, the macrophage, can come along and gobble the immune complex. Once you have been exposed to an invader, you will have antibodies on hand specifically targeted to that invader. Another encounter would be met with a swift response.

You may hear of substances called immunoglobulins. These are actually antibodies and are designated IgA (for immunoglobulin A), IgG, IgM, IgE, and IgD. Each have specific functions.

Natural killer cells. A final category of cell, the NK cells, is an independent sort of roving cell that kills viruses and cancer cells. It does not need to be signaled by T-cells, but carries out its work on its own.

The immune system is highly effective and has several redundant systems in case a part of it falters. Even so, many factors can interfere with immune function. Generally speaking, some of the key factors that influence the immune response are:

1. Diet and nutrition (food allergy/intolerance can lower immunity; nutritional insufficiency can lower immunity)
2. Genetics (certain genetic conditions are associated with sluggish immunity)
3. Lifestyle (exercise, smoking, etc.)
4. Environment (chemical exposure, etc.)
5. Psychological and social (stress, emotional suppression, attitude)

If you are fatigued, optimizing your immune response should be an integral part of your recovery program. The two primary steps in this are:

1. Reducing, eliminating, or avoiding factors that impair immunity.
2. Practicing or using methods that optimize immunity.

To discuss this would take an entire book. *Beyond Antibiotics* (North Atlantic Books, Berkeley, California) contains a discussion of a personal immune enhancement program, wherein I describe the aspects of diet, nutrition, lifestyle, environment, and psychology that can be modified to optimize your immune response.

In Review

1. Infection by bacteria, viruses, yeast, or parasites may contribute to fatigue.

2. Many such infections are chronic and not easily detected on a routine examination.

3. The symptoms may encompass many body systems including the respiratory tract, skin, brain and nervous system, endocrine system, digestive system, and immune system.

4. Laboratory tests are helpful in identifying if infection is present.

5. If infection is present, specific treatment is important.

6. Intestinal parasites should be considered as a possible cause of fatigue.

7. Along with specific treatment, address dietary, nutritional, lifestyle, environmental, and psychological factors that are known to optimize immunity.

Chapter 14

Antibiotic Overuse:
A Common Fatigue Trigger?

IN CHAPTER 13, I described how hidden infections may cause fatigue. In some of these cases, antibiotic treatment is appropriate and essential to recovery. However, antibiotics can sometimes be part of the problem and antibiotic *overuse* seems to be one important factor that gives rise to chronic fatigue. Recall the work of Carol Jessop, M.D., who reported that 88 percent of her chronic fatigue patients had a history of *recurrent antibiotic treatment* (as a child, adolescent or adult). Dr. William Crook, author of *Chronic Fatigue Syndrome and the Yeast Connection,* concludes similarly that the overuse of antibiotics is a major contributing factor to the development of chronic fatigue.[1] In a 1993 issue of *Preventive Medicine Update,* internist and pathologist Dr. Majid Ali reported that antibiotic overuse was a precipitating factor in about 80 percent of his patients with chronic fatigue.[2]

In 1991, Drs. David S. Bauman and Howard Hagglund reported in the *Journal of Advancement in Medicine* on a study of 43 women who were classified as "Polysystem Chronic Complainers." These were women who suffered from ten or more symptoms that included fatigue, poor memory, mood swings, head pressure, muscle aches, digestive symptoms and inability to concentrate. Of these 43 women, 29 (or 67 percent) reported having been on prolonged courses of antibiotics. Only five of 33 controls—reporting fewer than four complaints—had a history of prolonged antibiotic use.[3]

Beyond Antibiotics presents an extensive review of the problems associated with antibiotic overuse. One issue discussed was the emergence of more and more bacteria that are resistant to these drugs. When bacteria are able to resist antibiotics, the chance of life-threatening infection increases. In August 1992, officials from the Centers for Disease Control and Prevention and the National Institutes of Health sounded the alarm about the epidemic of antibiotic-resistant bacteria.[4]

Harold C. Neu, professor of medicine and pharmacology at Columbia University in New York, wrote a paper published in *Science* entitled "The Crisis in Antibiotic Resistance." In this article, he points out that in 1941, only 40,000 units of penicillin per day for four days were required to *cure* pneumococcal pneumonia. "Today," says Neu, "a patient could receive 24 million units of penicillin a day and die of pneumococcal meningitis." He adds that bacteria that cause infection of the respiratory tract, skin, bladder, bowel, and blood "...are now resistant to virtually all of the older antibiotics. The extensive use of antibiotics in the community and hospitals has fueled this crisis."[5]

A truly sobering chapter in the crisis of antibiotic resistance has begun to unfold. Many medical scientists now believe that antibiotics may be a crucial cofactor in the development of AIDS. Proponents of this hypothesis include some of the most prominent names in the field. Included are Dr. Luc Montagnier, director of virology at the Pasteur Institute in France and discoverer of the HIV virus; Dr. Peter Duseberg, professor of molecular biology and virology at the University of California at Berkeley, and one of the world's foremost authorities on retroviruses; Dr. Robert Root-Bernstein, professor of immunology and physiology, University of Michigan; and Dr. Jeffrey Fisher, consultant to the World Health Organization and author of *The Plague Makers*.[6]

These and other scientists warn that the overuse of antibiotics may contribute to the immune collapse of people in high-risk groups and increase the risk to untreatable secondary infections. They contend that overuse of antibiotics has created a situation for which there is no parallel in human history.

A common consequence of antibiotic overuse is disruption of the normal balance of intestinal bacteria. The intestinal tract is home to billions of normal bacteria that help us by synthesizing vitamins, digesting certain foodstuffs and toxins, and protecting our guts from infection by parasites, bacteria, and viruses. Most people are shocked to learn that organisms living in the *healthy* intestinal tract outnumber our total body cells by ten times. It is well known that antibiotics, especially broad-spectrum antibiotics, can eliminate not only the harmful bacteria for which they are intended, but beneficial bacteria as well. Once these drugs reach the intestinal tract, they eliminate helpful bacteria and may lead to overgrowth of yeast and other harmful organisms in the gut.

For example, we know yeast is used to ferment sugar into alcohol. This is the fundamental principle that has allowed the development of beer and wine for centuries. The human gut is no different. If you have overgrowth of yeast, dietary sugars can be converted into alcohol. Recent studies have shown that in people with chronic health problems, 65 percent were found to convert dietary sugar into alcohol, which was then absorbed into the bloodstream. In some cases, the blood alcohol rose to levels that would have declared the people legally drunk. This phenomenon has been called "the auto-brewery syndrome."[7]

Nutritional status becomes especially important in such cases. For instance, patients who have insufficient zinc in their bodies do not adequately detoxify alcohol because the enzyme is zinc-dependent. This can further aggravate the problem of the person with dysbiosis.

The problem of dysbiosis is compounded in certain people because some of these bacteria and yeast cause the production of aldehydes in the body. Formaldehyde is one form of aldehyde. Aldehydes can be terribly toxic to the body, including the nervous system. The effect can be fatigue, nervous system symptoms, liver stress, and more. In people who have insufficient levels of the trace element molybdenum (which is somewhat common in chronically ill people), the enzyme that detoxifies aldehydes (aldehyde oxidase) is not fully active. The aldehydes are then converted into a toxic nervous system chemical called chloral hydrate, or what used to be known as "knock-out drops." Molybdenum insufficiency is made more likely by the poor mineral absorption that has been caused by antibiotic overuse and yeast/bacterial overgrowth in the gut. You can see how a vicious cycle is set in motion by antibiotic overuse.

aldehyde/toxin production
Antibiotics → yeast/bacteria overgrowth → poor absorption → vitamin/mineral insufficiency → poor detoxification → chronic fatigue

Dysbiosis, or overgrowth of microbes in the gut, takes four basic forms according to Leo Galland, M.D. They are:[8]

1. *Putrefactive.* This form of dysbiosis results from diets high in fat and animal fiber. The gut microbes putrefy, or digest, the food materials and convert them into toxins. These toxins come in contact with the gut cells and can be absorbed into the body. These chemical products of bacterial putrefaction have been associated with some cases of colon and breast cancer. The gut bacteria can also influence hormone levels such as estrogen.

2. *Fermentation excess.* This form of dysbiosis is due to the bacterial fermentation of carbohydrates and sugars. Common symptoms include fatigue, malaise, flatulence, diarrhea, constipation, and abdominal distension. People with this form of dysbiosis often do not tolerate fiber well. They also may convert dietary sugar into alcohol, which is then absorbed into the bloodstream.

3. *Deficiency.* Excessive antibiotic exposure or inadequate fiber intake can lead to a general decrease in the normal microbes that should live in a healthy gut. For this condition, a substance called fructooligosaccharides (FOS) is often given to stimulate growth of the normal gut microbes.

4. *Sensitization.* More research is beginning to show that disruption of the normal gut flora can lead to inflammatory diseases of the gut and to autoimmune disorders. Autoimmune disorders are con-

ditions in which the immune system attacks one's own body. Examples are lupus, thyroiditis, and some forms of arthritis.

A doctor who is trained to recognize the important role of the intestinal tract in chronic illness can truly be an asset in your effort to uncover the causes of fatigue and low vitality.

Signs and Symptoms

The signs and symptoms must be associated with a history of chronic antibiotic use as a child, adolescent, or adult. Large doses of antibiotics over a short period of time may also lead to similar problems. Chronic gastrointestinal complaints are common. Fatigue is a hallmark sign.

Laboratory Tests

Because of the widespread disruption that can occur as a result of antibiotic overuse, there are few specific tests that can be recommended. You doctor will likely run tests that are appropriate for your particular complaint. One test that may be of value to assess the status of the intestinal tract (which is often hardest hit by antibiotic overuse) is the Comprehensive Digestive Stool Analysis (CDSA) performed by Great Smokies Diagnostic Laboratory (Asheville, North Carolina). This is a stool test that evaluates 24 different parameters of intestinal function such as absorption and digestion of fat, vegetables, and meat protein, and the presence of bacterial or yeast overgrowth. The test sample is stool, or feces, as the name implies. Below is a list of the parameters tested.[9]

Triglycerides	Chymotrypsin
Vegetable fibers	Long chain fatty acids
Short-chain fatty acids	Bacteria
Cholesterol	Meat fibers
Yeast/fungi	

- Urinary organic acids for microbial metabolites
- Intestinal permeability test (lactulose/mannitol)
- Breath hydrogen/methane

If you have a history of antibiotic overuse, gastrointestinal complaints, chronic fatigue, or other chronic symptoms, these tests can be a valuable first step. Remember, you can take all the vitamins and minerals in the world, but if your intestinal tract is out of balance and absorbing poorly, or worse, producing toxins, you will not improve until the intestinal problems are corrected.

Treatment

Treatment of someone with chronic fatigue who has a history of antibiotic overuse is often complicated. It is certainly beyond the scope of this book. Every effort should be made to find means to improve immunity and reduce the need for antibiotic therapy. This may seem like an ominous task, but many of the steps have been outlined in *Beyond Antibiotics.*[10]

Probiotics are being used by many holistic doctors to treat those with a history of dysbiosis or chronic antibiotic therapy. Probiotics consist of substances designed to restore balance to the microbial population of the intestinal tract. Usually this means acidophilus, bifidus, *S. faecium,* and other organisms. It may also mean agents that promote growth of these helpful organisms like fructooligosaccharides and antibody complexes from whey. Fructooligosaccharides are starch-like materials that promote the growth of bifidobacteria, an important beneficial microbe of the gut. Antibody complexes from whey include a product known as Inner Strength, which helps the body fight intestinal infections by viruses, yeast, and other organisms.

If you have suffered from chronic fatigue, tiredness, and low vitality, and if you have a history of chronic antibiotic use, you must approach your problem somewhat differently than a person who does not have this history. The areas you must consider addressing include:

- *Food allergy or food intolerance.* Identify foods to which you are sensitive and reduce the antigen (allergen) load.
- *Nutritional insufficiency.* Identify nutrient insufficiencies that exist and replenish appropriate nutrients.

- *Candida overgrowth and dysbiosis of the gut.* Identify whether yeast overgrowth has occurred and the balance of normal gut bacteria such as *L. acidophilus, B. bifidum, E. coli,* etc. A special diet and antifungal medication (or botanical) may be necessary. Probiotics may be necessary.
- *Leaky gut syndrome.* Test for excessive gut permeability and supply nutrients that help to repair the gut lining.
- *Absorption problems.* Digestion of food may be impaired. Determine if enzymes of digestion are being properly secreted and if food is being properly broken down. Supply digestive aids if needed.
- *Immunological problems.* All of the above can contribute to faulty immune regulation and repair.
- *Chemical sensitivity (possibly).* Some patients with a history of antibiotic overuse, dysbiosis, candida overgrowth, and food allergy develop sensitivity to perfumes and other odors. This must be dealt with as well.

In Review

1. Antibiotic overuse can contribute to the development of chronic fatigue.
2. Those with a history of antibiotic overuse often suffer from disrupted intestinal ecology that contributes to poor digestive function, food intolerance, leaky gut, or other problems.
3. The problems of antibiotic overuse must be addressed by rebuilding intestinal bacteria and restoring optimum intestinal function.
4. Those with a history of antibiotic overuse should attempt to reduce their reliance on antibiotics by focusing on ways to optimize immunity. This includes focusing on diet, nutrition, lifestyle, environment, and psychological factors.
5. Acidophilus and bifidus supplements should be considered when there is a history of antibiotic overuse.

Chapter 15

Cancer, Heart Disease, Lung Disease, and Other Chronic Conditions

FATIGUE IS ONE of the major symptoms in early cardiovascular disease, cancer, and lung disease. Other disease categories in which fatigue may be a primary complaint are neurological diseases, circulatory disorders, endocrine diseases, kidney disease, and autoimmune diseases. In some cases, fatigue may be the only sign that these conditions exist. It is beyond the scope of this book to discuss all the signs and ramifications of these disorders since the list is so long. It would look like a recreation of a medical textbook.

Since fatigue is a primary complaint in numerous diseases, it is important that you not merely assume your fatigue is due to vitamin or mineral deficiency, insomnia, allergies, or many of the others factors discussed in this book. Have your doctor do a complete physical to make sure these more serious causes of fatigue are ruled out.

Below is just a partial list of some serious medical conditions that can contribute to fatigue.

Chronic hepatitis	Myasthenia gravis
Multiple sclerosis	Addison's disease
Cushing's syndrome	Advanced diabetes mellitus
Alcoholism	Kidney disease

Hematological disease	AIDS
Lupus	Sarcoidosis
Endocarditis	Occult abscess
Histoplasmosis	Schizophrenia
Anxiety neurosis	Malignancy of any organ or
Congestive heart	tissue
Blood clots	Occlusive vascular disease
Emphysema	

If you have a family history of any of these diseases it is especially important that your case be carefully investigated.

While such disease states are often serious and debilitating, they can also be responsive to changes in lifestyle, improvement in nutrition, behavioral therapy, detoxification, exercise, and other forms of medicine that use an integrated approach. Do not assume that just because you have a "medical diagnosis" that you are relegated to living with your condition. The practices of holistic doctors and allopathic doctors are full of people who have made recoveries from illness for which there was said to be "no cure."

In 1986, a 60-year-old, severely fatigued man named Walter came to my clinic with nephrotic syndrome, a serious disease of the kidneys. He had been told that he had only six months to live and that there was little else his doctors could do. The pitting edema in his legs was so severe that when I pressed my finger into his ankle the half-inch depression was detectable for about five minutes. I made him no promises whatsoever, but suggested that if he made some very substantial changes we might improve the quality of his remaining months.

Walter was a farmer from Wisconsin who had worked with agricultural chemicals much of his life, and I suspected this might be in part responsible for his kidney failure. I recommended a detoxification program (which at that time was not as sophisticated as we have today), homeopathic medicines, antioxidant nutrients, a low-allergen diet, and some psychological techniques and behavioral changes.

He remained on the program for about six months. To the surprise of Walter, his family, and myself his condition improved dramatically. His specialists were astounded that he was in such remarkable condition considering the unfavorable prognosis. Two years later he was admitted to the hospital with an unrelated heart incident. At that time, his doctors expressed further astonishment that the heart incident had not caused his kidneys to fail. Walter lived several years longer after which I moved and lost touch with him. This man's recovery was quite rewarding to me. It was an affirmation of what's possible in the face of what seem to be incredible odds.

Laboratory Tests

The diseases discussed in this chapter span the entire spectrum of medical diagnosis and could involve almost any known test. Practically speaking, your doctor will probably begin with a standard SMAC, a thyroid panel, lipid panel, sed rate, and urinalysis. He or she would then move on to whatever test was indicated based on your symptoms and history.

Treatment

Treatment will be directed at the specific condition present. In general, I believe any serious disease requires that one also consider the following factors:

- Careful assessment and treatment directed at diet and nutrition.
- Appropriate alterations in lifestyle, such as exercise.
- Consideration of environmental factors.
- Use of psychological and behavioral techniques to enhance recovery.

In Review

1. Chronic fatigue can be one of the primary symptoms of cancer, heart disease, lung disease, nervous system disease, kidney disease, and other conditions.

2. If you suffer from fatigue of unknown origin, see your
   doctor for a physical (and appropriate tests if necessary).

3. Many chronic illnesses can be helped by modifying diet,
   lifestyle, and attitude, in addition to taking specific
   treatment measures. In fact, chronic illness is more
   responsive to an integrated approach than to a solely
   pharmaceutical approach.

Chapter 16

Prescription Drugs That Make You Tired

MANY COMMONLY USED prescription and non-prescription drugs can produce fatigue. If you suffer from fatigue and are taking medication of any kind, the first question you should ask is "Is fatigue a known side effect of my medication?"

William was a 55-year-old businessman with high blood pressure. He was constantly on the go and worked 15-hour days. Remarkably, he seemed to have the stamina to work this hard and truly enjoyed what he was doing. The problem arose when he began taking Reserpine for his hypertension. He became sluggish, tired, and fell asleep in the middle of conversations—not only when listening but also when he was the speaker! He was unable to work his normal schedule and felt tired throughout his working day. When his medication was changed, his fatigue improved. His new medication was less of a problem, but still induced some fatigue. His fatigue completely cleared when diet and nutritional therapy were used to manage his hypertension.

Joan was on Inderal, a beta-blocker, for what her doctors believed was mitral valve prolapse. The Inderal caused her to be so tired she could barely care for her family. One of her doctors thought she had narcolepsy, a disorder where one simply falls asleep in the middle of activity. It is not a good idea to stop Inderal abruptly, so Joan was placed on coenzyme Q_{10}, carnitine, essential fatty acids, magnesium, taurine, and some other nutrients. Gradually her sleepiness and mitral valve symptoms improved. Her heart condition improved enough to be taken off the medication and her fatigue fully disappeared.

Richard Podell, M.D., author of *Doctor, Why Am I So Tired?*, has compiled a list of the top 150 prescription drugs in the United States and listed the fatigue-inducing potential of each one on a scale from zero to three. Of these 150 drugs, 109 are listed as having the potential, either directly or indirectly, to cause fatigue. Some cause severe fatigue, some only minor fatigue.[1] Jesse Stoff, M.D., has treated several thousand patients with chronic fatigue and is the author of *Chronic Fatigue Syndrome: The Hidden Epidemic.* He also contends that prescription drugs are an important cause of fatigue that must be ruled out.[2]

The most common categories of drugs that cause fatigue are:

1. Antihypertensives
2. Antidepressants
3. Tranquilizers
4. Sleeping pills
5. Antihistamines
6. Antibiotics (when used extensively over time)
7. Diuretics
8. Illicit drugs
9. Alcohol

One means by which prescription drugs may contribute to fatigue is by causing nutrient deficiencies. For example, diuretics cause loss of potassium and magnesium, which can lead to fatigue. Dilantin and phenobarbital can cause deficiency of folic acid, which we earlier saw can lead to fatigue. Chronic use of aspirin can lead to loss of folic acid and iron, development of leaky gut syndrome, fatigue, and food allergies.[3,4]

The high blood pressure medication, hydralazine, is a vitamin B_6 antagonist. Use of cimetidine (Tagamet) to treat ulcers can lead to deficiency of B_{12}. Some drugs, such as tricyclic antidepressants, may adversely influence appetite. Others can cause malabsorption and lead to poor uptake of nutrients.[5]

Prescription drugs can also add to the toxic burden themselves and strain the elimination mechanisms of the body. Some drugs, like Seldane, adversely affect the liver's ability to detoxify foreign chemicals (by blocking an enzyme system known as the mixed function oxidase system).[6] Such an event occurred in 1992 when a Dallas man became quite sick while taking Tagamet (which also blocks the liver's detoxifying mechanism) and subsequently was exposed to lawn chemicals.

According to neurologist Dr. Stewart Tepper, many patients suffer from "chronic tension-type headaches," "rebound headaches," or "drug-induced refractory headaches syndrome." He has found that these types of headaches are related to toxicity symptoms. Many such patients are on pain relievers such as aspirin or acetaminophen, even though the drugs provide no symptomatic relief. Dr. Tepper points out that these drugs, in quantities as small as ten tablets per week, can cause chronic headache syndrome because they interfere with the liver's normal detoxication mechanisms.[7]

Drugs may also contribute to symptoms of fatigue because they contain coloring, additives, and preservatives to which an individual may be sensitive. Many drugs, for example, contain sulfites, which may adversely affect asthmatics. The food colorings yellow #5 and yellow #6 are widely used in the manufacture of drugs and cause adverse reactions in certain hypersensitive patients.

Many doctors are not aware of the adverse nutritional and other consequences of the drugs they prescribe. For this reason, you may have to do your homework or consult with a nutrition-oriented doctor.

If you suffer from fatigue or low energy, and are on prescription drugs, consider the possibility that the drug may be a cause. If your doctor does not adequately address the issue, look up the name of your medication in a *Physician's Desk Reference* (at your public library) and check if fatigue is listed as a complication.[8] Quite often, fatigue is not listed as a symptom if it has not occurred in a high percentage of people. However, it may still affect you. *Doctor, Why Am I So Tired?* also contains a good summary of the fatigue-causing prescription drugs.[9]

Talk with your pharmacist and ask if the medication you are on can cause fatigue as a side effect. If he or she answers "yes," ask which other medication might serve the same purpose without inducing fatigue. Ultimately, your doctor will have to make the change in prescription since the pharmacist cannot do this. But you will have the information you need to go to your doctor.

Signs and Symptoms

Prescription drugs can trigger symptoms in almost any body system. Fatigue, tiredness, and low vitality are among these.

Laboratory Tests

There are no standard laboratory tests to determine if medication is causing your fatigue. You and your doctor can make the determination by asking questions such as:

1. When did I start taking the drug?
2. When was the onset of my fatigue symptoms?
3. Are the fatigue symptoms associated with beginning the drug?

The determining test is whether your fatigue symptoms improve after changing or discontinuing the drug. Since many drugs adversely affect vitamin or mineral levels, laboratory tests to assess nutrient status may be necessary. See chapter 27 for a description of these tests. In addition, tests of liver function are important when taking drugs such as ketoconazole, Seldane, Tagamet, and many others.

Treatment

The standard treatment for fatigue that is associated with prescription drugs is to change or discontinue the medication. This should only be done under your doctor's supervision.

Any nutrient deficiencies that occur as a result of drug therapy should also be addressed. This also should be done under a doctor's supervision, since some nutrients interfere with drug action.

In Review

1. Prescription drugs are an important cause of fatigue.

2. Certain drugs have a greater capacity to induce fatigue than others.

3. Some drugs do not directly cause fatigue by themselves, but may in combination with others.

4. Some drugs alter vitamin or mineral status.

5. Some drugs, such as Seldane, impair the liver's ability to detoxify foreign chemicals encountered in the environment.

6. If you are fatigued you should take a careful look at your medication history. See your doctor. If he is unwilling to take a serious look at the matter, consult the PDR and see if the drug you are taking can contribute to fatigue. If so, return to your doctor with this information.

7. Do not stop taking a medication without your doctor's orders. Abruptly stopping some medication can be dangerous.

Chapter 17

Tired or Toxic?

THE ENVIRONMENTAL PROTECTION AGENCY (EPA) currently recognizes more than four million chemical compounds. More than 60,000 of these are produced commercially, with three new compounds introduced each day. In 1992, the EPA published the results of a study in which the urine of 7,000 randomly sampled Americans was tested for toxic chemical residues. Chemicals like pentachlorophenol, a wood preservative, and others were found in 71 percent of individuals tested. These were not people working at chemical factories or industrial waste incinerators. This study looked at the average citizen—you and me.[1] It is disconcerting to find such a high percentage of individuals with chemical residue in their urine. These are all chemicals not even in existence 100 years ago.

Many doctors who work with chronically fatigued patients and those who work in the field of environmental medicine agree that chemical exposure is a major contributor to fatigue and low vitality. For example, if you review the symptoms of formaldehyde exposure you will find fatigue, depression, and poor concentration right at the top. The symptoms of exposure to trichloroethylene (found in floor polish, copy machines, carpet cleaner, etc.) include fatigue, poor concentration, and drowsiness, among others.[2] Exposure to toluene, the most common indoor air pollutant, triggers symptoms of fatigue, poor concentration, drowsiness, and headache.

Methylene chloride is found in paint thinner, hair spray, adhesives, paint, solvents, flame-retardents, and many other common products. The aerosol propellants found in hair sprays, antiperspirants, air fresheners, and spray paint may contain up to 50 percent methylene chloride. Once inhaled, methylene chloride goes directly to the brain, fat cells, and liver. Common symptoms include fatigue, lethargy, headaches, and chest pain.[3]

In an article entitled "Chronic Fatigue Syndrome and Chemical Overload," Dr. R. A. Buist explained that there are many pieces of evidence suggesting that chronic fatigue may be a result of toxin exposure. He goes on to point out that toxins can disrupt muscle metabolism, accounting for the pain and fatigability of muscles experienced by many fatigued people. Buist also notes that in many chronic fatigue patients, use of recreational drugs or environmental exposure preceded the onset of their fatigue.[4]

In an address to the Well Mind Association in Seattle, Washington, David S. Buscher, M.D., made the following remarks: "My personal theory on chronic fatigue is that the increased load of pollutants in our environment, such as pesticides, is causing people to have a breakdown of their immune systems ... I would say 70 percent of my patients with chronic fatigue had a chemical trigger; they moved into a new home, there was remodeling at the office, or a pesticide application, and now they have chronic fatigue. I think the mechanism is some kind of cellular poisoning from these chemicals. The affected person's detoxication* system is clogged up or destroyed, they get a backlog of chemicals, and their immune system goes down."[5]

In 1992, the neurobehavioral effects of various chemicals were reviewed in *Environmental Neurotoxicity*, published by the National Research Council. The following symptoms commonly associated with fatigue and the number of chemicals that may cause these symptoms are significant.[6]

---

*The term *detoxication* is often used to described the body's system of processing toxic substances. The term *detoxification* is used to describe therapy aimed at removing toxic substances that have accumulated in the body.

Symptom	Number of Chemicals
Fatigue	87
Listlessness	30
Depression	40
Sleep disturbances	119
Weakness	179

An important fact about chemical exposure is the role that cumulative exposure plays in causing illness. Exposure to trace amounts of one chemical may produce few ill effects. However, when five, ten, or ever fifty different compounds are encountered in trace amounts, which is not unusual, the additive effects can be serious. To put this in perspective, consider that in one Washington, D.C., home for the elderly, 350 different volatile chemicals were found in the indoor air.[7] Another study conducted by the EPA found anywhere from 40 to 120 different organic compounds circulating in the air of every home tested, regardless of whether the home was in urban Chicago or rural North Dakota.[8]

In an analysis of the exhaled breath of suburban New Jersey residents, researchers detected chloroform, trichloroethane, benzene, styrene, xylene, carbon tetrachloride, dichlorobenzene, ethyl benzene, trichloroethylene, and other compounds.[9] It doesn't take a chemist to know that these chemicals do not belong in the body. However, it does take a doctor with sufficient knowledge of biochemistry to figure out what to do about this problem when illness results.

Chemical toxins affect individuals in vastly different ways, depending upon their individual biochemical make-up. There are several key factors that determine how an individual will react to chemical exposure.

1. *Nutritional status.* Vitamins, minerals, amino acids, and other nutrient factors play a vital role in detoxication of foreign chemicals.

2. *Total toxic load.* The amount of toxin, the number of toxins, and the duration of exposure to toxins determine health effects.

3. *Genetics.* Due to genetic deficiencies or abnormalities of certain enzymes, some individuals do not detoxify as readily.

4. *Age.* Children are more susceptible than adults.

5. *State of health.* Someone with chronic illness, liver disease, or altered immunity may be less able to adequately detoxify.

6. *Stress.*

7. *Immune system status.* Some reactions to toxins are mediated by the immune system.

Your nutritional status has everything to do with how your detoxication systems work and how you handle the toxins in your environment. If you are deficient in the trace element molybdenum, an enzyme called aldehyde oxidase does not function properly. Under these circumstances, if you were exposed to a common pollutant such as formaldehyde, it would not be properly detoxified. In fact, such compounds are shunted into another pathway that forms other, often more toxic, compounds. In the case of formaldehyde, it gets converted into chloral hydrate—also known as a "Mickey Finn" or "knockout drops." The effect is a dopey, foggy, fatigued feeling, like you were drunk, but without the euphoria.[10] If you are deficient in magnesium many aspects of the detoxication mechanism do not work. The same is true of zinc deficiency.

In one of your body's detoxication pathways, toxic substances are temporarily converted into *more* toxic intermediate substances and then converted into mercapturic acids to be harmlessly eliminated. However, if you are deficient in vitamin E, selenium, glutathione, glycine, vitamin C, or other nutrients, the highly toxic intermediates are not properly quenched and can wreak considerable havoc with your cells.

The immune system can become seriously impaired by exposure to chemicals. Some chemical exposures may act to suppress immunity, while others may cause the immune system to overreact. The former circumstance leads to susceptibility to infections and perhaps cancer. The latter leads to autoimmune diseases in which the immune system attacks the body's own cells. Some arthritic conditions, lupus, and some thyroid disorders are examples of this latter effect.

In a study published in the *Archives of Environmental Health,* people who were exposed to chlordane, used to control termites, had immune system defects that were detectable up to *ten years* after the exposure.[11] Other studies show the devastating effect of chemicals on immune function. Thus, toxicity not only directly causes fatigue, but can render us more susceptible to bacterial and viral infection, both of which are common causes of persistent fatigue.

In 1990, Sherry Rogers, M.D., wrote a book entitled *Tired or Toxic?* in which she describes in great detail how toxicity contributes to fatigue. She mentions that the most common organ affected by chemical exposure is the brain, leading to drowsiness, fatigue, exhaustion, sluggish thinking, or a host of other symptoms. She states, "Frequently, most of these people are initially too intimidated and embarrassed to mention how exhausted they are. Instead they concentrate on the more visible symptoms that can be more readily verified. Medicine, unfortunately, delegates brain symptoms ... to the psychiatrists."[12]

One means by which chemicals may contribute to fatigue is by affecting thyroid function, a common cause of low vitality. Chlorinated compounds are well known for their effects on thyroid function. Many of these compete directly with thyroid hormones or proteins that carry thyroid hormones. One such chemical, pentachlorophenol, was found to significantly lower the level of both the active and inactive form of thyroid hormone.[13]

Chemicals may also interfere with sleep, leading to chronic fatigue. Sixty-six men exposed to solvents on the job were assessed for sleep apnea. Sleep apnea is a disorder of interrupted breathing during sleep that leaves many sufferers chronically tired. Sleep apnea occurred in roughly one-fifth of the men, which prompted the investigators to conclude that some cases of sleep apnea may be solvent-induced encephalopathy.[14] In 112 individuals evaluated for exposure to organic solvents (house paints, spray finishers, printing), there was a significantly higher prevalence of insomnia.[15] In *Environmental Neurotoxicology,* it is reported that any one of 119 different chemicals can cause sleep disturbance.[16]

Because of the pervasive use of chemicals in our society, a new disease has emerged known as multiple chemical sensitivity (MCS). While chemical exposure affects all of us to one degree or another, people with MCS are severely affected. People with chemical sensitivity often become ill from being in the presence of only minute amounts of a chemical. To them, a faint odor of formaldehyde can cause devastating symptoms of fatigue. Unfortunately, others around them who cannot smell the odors label them as hypochondriacs, often noting, "If I can't smell it you must be imagining it." This is far from the truth, and chemically sensitive people can take some comfort in the fact that the health effects of low level chemical exposure are becoming more documentable.

For example, Dr. Donald Dudley, at the Washington Institute of Neurosciences in Seattle, found that when patients were exposed to chemicals to which they reported sensitivity, they showed significant changes in their visual and auditory evoked potential readings—a measure of the rate at which nerves transmit messages from the eyes and ears to the brain.[17] Gary Schwartz, Ph.D., and his research team at the University of Arizona showed that the brain registers exposure to a chemical odor even though the nose does not sense its presence.[18] Russell Jaffe, M.D., of Reston, Virginia, has demonstrated that a variety of immune reactions to chemicals occur in people with chronic illness.[19]

Toxic minerals are another important cause of fatigue in some people. Included are lead, mercury, cadmium, arsenic, aluminum, nickel, silver, beryllium, and tin. Recall the interview with Dr. Majid Ali who estimated that roughly 40 percent of his patients with chronic fatigue suffer from heavy metal toxicity. He observed that aluminum toxicity was most common, with lead and mercury toxicity not far behind.[20] Aluminum toxicity would be expected to cause fatigue because it blocks the major energy molecule in the body, ATP. Lead and mercury impair immune function, block enzyme function, impair memory and nervous system function, trigger the release of inflammatory substances, and alter certain metabolic pathways.

Researchers at Upssala University Medical School in Sweden reported that patients with chronic fatigue contain abnormal levels of mercury within their cells.[21] Another group tested sensitivity to metals such as lead and mercury using a method of testing known as MELISA (Memory Lymphocyte Immuno Stimulation Assay). Of patients with chronic fatigue, 45 percent showed mercury hypersensitivity and 49 percent showed lead hypersensitivity. When the metal burden was removed from the body (in many cases by removing mercury-containing silver dental fillings), 77 percent of patients reported improved health.[22]

Signs and Symptoms

The symptoms of chemical toxicity are far too numerous to mention. In general, chemical exposure affects different people in different ways, depending on their individual biochemistry, nutritional status, stress levels, level of exposure, and many other factors. Conditions ranging from thyroid disease, cardiovascular disease, kidney disease, endocrine diseases, depression, psychosis, and many other disorders can be triggered or caused by chemical exposure or toxicity.

Fatigue, sluggishness, and low energy are among the most common symptoms of toxicity. If you experience these symptoms and your health problems seem to defy identification or do not respond to treatment, it may be that you are ill because of toxicity. Certainly, those who work in occupations where chemicals are used should be screened for toxicity. However, many people who have no contact with industrial chemicals whatsoever experience exposure that seriously impairs their health.

Laboratory Tests

Below are a number of tests that can be used to determine if you suffer from toxic exposure, if your detoxication system is working or overloaded, if you have immune reactivity to environmental chemicals, if you have adequate antioxidant capacity, and if you have fatty tissue damage. To run all of these tests would be quite expensive. Most doctors working in environmental medicine would likely choose specific tests based your individual circumstances. This list shows the varied tests that are available to any doctor who wishes to do more detective work.

- *Urinary D-glucaric acid.* Helps determine if toxic exposure has taken place or whether your detoxication system is working properly.
- *Urinary mercapturic acid.* A byproduct of one of the body's detoxication pathways. Determines if toxic exposure has taken place.
- *Whole blood glutathione or glutathione peroxidase.* Shows the levels of an important nutrient involved in detoxication and its functional enzyme.
- *Total lipid peroxides.* Shows whether the lipids (or fats) that comprise your cell membranes are being damaged by free radicals.
- *Formic acid.* Shows whether your body is able to detoxify aldehydes such as formaldehyde.
- *ELISA/ACT.* A blood test that looks at delayed immune system reactivity to various substances including foreign chemicals, food allergens, food additives, molds, pollens, etc.
- *Amino acid analysis.* Assesses many aspects of metabolism and function. Shows amino acid deficiencies, and vitamin and mineral deficiencies.
- *Organic acid analysis.* Measures aspects of energy metabolism.
- *Serum and red blood cell vitamins and minerals.*
- *Provocation-neutralization test.* Done in a physician's office, this test determines sensitivity to chemicals and identifies a neutralizing dose that can be helpful in reducing symptoms.
- *Hair mineral analysis.* Assesses level of toxic metals and some trace elements. Other tests used to test for toxic metals include:
  - Whole blood heavy element. Assesses toxic minerals in blood.
  - RBC or WBC heavy element. Assesses toxic minerals in cells.
  - Urine or post-challenge urine. Challenge substance, such as DMPS (dimercaptopropane sulfate) is given to purge metals from body, which can then be measured in urine.
  - MELISA (Memory Lymphocyte Immuno Stimulation Assay). Assesses immune reactivity to metals.

• *Blood levels of toxic substances* such as benzene, toluene, and others.

A beginning laboratory panel that one might consider to assess toxicity might include:[23]

Mercapturic acid	D-glucaric acid
Formic acid	Glutathione peroxidase
Lipid peroxides	

Treatment

Toxicity is a very complicated phenomenon that requires the guidance of a doctor trained in environmental medicine and nutritional biochemistry. Toxic mineral exposure is treated differently than exposure to organic chemical compounds. Specific nutrients are necessary to enhance biochemical detoxication pathways of the body. Any recommendations made in this book could only be considered superficial and general. When dealing with toxicity problems, the following areas must be addressed:

1. Reduce the total toxic load by removing toxins from your environment and by removing offending foods and additives from your diet.
2. Identify functional nutrient deficiencies related to detoxication and general metabolism.
3. Restore your body's pH to its normal balance so that cellular systems begin to function normally.
4. Begin a supervised detoxification program aimed at removing toxins stored in body tissues.

Nutrients important in detoxification include:

L-glutathione	Vitamin E
Vitamin C	*N*-acetylcysteine
Selenium	Beta-carotene
Coenzyme Q_{10}	Taurine
Zinc	Copper
Magnesium	Molybdenum
Bioflavonoids	

5. Utilize a low temperature sauna. Some doctors who treat patients with toxic exposure recommend that patients sit in a low temperature sauna for several hours each day. The low temperature encourages a "fat sweat" to eliminate toxins that are stored in the body's fat.

6. Support the endocrine, immune, and hepatic (liver) system.

7. Begin a program of behavioral therapy and stress management.

8. Restore gastrointestinal function.

In Review

1. Our environment is filled with chemicals to which we are exposed.

2. Each of us reacts uniquely to exposure based on our biochemical individuality.

3. Chemical exposure, be it great or small, can disrupt the body's metabolism and lead to fatigue or many other syndromes.

4. Chemical exposure can significantly affect nutritional status, which further impairs the body's ability to deal with toxic substances in the future.

5. Nutritional supplementation is essential to restore normal metabolic balance in anyone who suffers from multiple chemical sensitivity, or who has suffered from chemical toxicity that impairs health.

6. Detoxification programs that attempt to lower the body's level of toxic substances are an important means of improving health.

7. Toxic metals can contribute to fatigue. They do so by interfering with brain function, enzymes, immune function, energy production, and by other means. Included are aluminum, mercury, lead, cadmium, arsenic, nickel, tin, and others.

8. Common nutrients protect against heavy metal toxicity.

9. Hair, urine, and blood can be used to determine if heavy metal toxicity is present.

10. Nutrients can be used to chelate or remove heavy metals from the body. However, in serious cases intravenous use of a chelating substance must be applied.

11. Toxicity can affect anyone.

Suggested Reading

If you would like more information about environmental toxicity and health effects obtain a copy of *Tired or Toxic* by Sherry Rogers, M.D. (Prestige Publishing, Syracuse, New York, 1990). For health professionals interested in a textbook of environmental medicine obtain the four-part series by William Rea, M.D. entitled *Chemical Sensitivity* (Lewis Publishers, Boca Raton, Florida, 1993.)

Chapter 18

Airborne Allergy

MANY PEOPLE WHO suffer from fatigue do so as a result of airborne substances. It may also be due to climatic factors. The most common airborne substances are:

1. *Mold and fungi.* Sensitivity to mold or fungi is a very common, yet often undiagnosed problem. Sherry Rogers, M.D., who works extensively with chronically ill patients, claims that many of her fatigued patients have sensitivity to molds that are not routinely tested for.[1]

Carol's case illustrates this point. She had been experiencing chronic muscle pain, bouts of fatigue, insomnia, nervousness, rapid heart beat, confusion, and memory loss. She noted that symptoms were worse in the summer months, though still present in winter. In certain areas of the house she felt especially ill. She felt better when up at the lake home. We placed special plates designed to detect mold in the basement, bedroom, and living room of her primary residence. The results were very interesting. High mold counts were found in each of the areas tested, although different types were found in different locations. Spores found included:

Cladosporium	Acremonium
Epicoccum	Aureobasidium
Penicillium	Rhodotorula
Moniliaceous, sterile fungi	Pitheuyces

Of the above molds, she had more than eight colony counts, which is significant. Her IgE blood tests also revealed sensitivity to mold. This was more than enough to suggest she had significant environmental problems that had to be addressed before her health would improve.

A similar case is noteworthy. Terry had moved into an upstairs office of a stylish old home. Not long after working in his new environment, Terry began to suffer from fatigue and a chronic cough. The symptoms gradually became quite debilitating. A mold plate sampling of his office revealed cladosporium, alternaria, and moniliaceous sterile fungi. The cladosporium colony count alone was 12! His total colony count was 16. No wonder he was having problems. A total colony count over seven is considered indicative of serious environmental problems. His office contained more than twice that threshold.

2. *Pollens, grasses, animals.* Pollen and grass allergies tend to be very seasonal in nature. If you are fatigued in the summer months, but not during winter, you may be sensitive to pollens or grasses. This can be checked using a blood test such as the ELISA/ACT or IgE RAST.

For some years, Rick could not understand his cyclical bouts of fatigue throughout the summer. Three times each summer he would be leveled by his tiredness. Each period lasted about two weeks. We discovered he was allergic to alfalfa. Farmers cut hay three times each summer. The cutting, drying, and baling process lasted about two to three weeks for each cutting.

Another patient, Annie, suffered from fatigue, a rash, and chronically congested lungs. We finally traced the problem to her pet cockatoo. She sent the bird off to her sister's house for a while and her symptoms cleared up.

3. *Outdoor chemical pollutants.* Pollution in large cities is a growing problem. Chemicals such as ozone, sulfur dioxide, carbon monoxide, nitrogen dioxide, and organic chemicals cause substantial chemical stress on our bodies. Some chemicals can cause fatigue directly, while others cause it indirectly. Carbon monoxide, for example, competes with oxygen on the hemoglobin molecules carried by

red blood cells. If our red cells don't carry enough oxygen we become, tired, sluggish, and easily fatigued. Other chemicals, like ozone and petrochemical hydrocarbons, produce oxidative stress that uses up more of our antioxidant nutrients.

4. *Indoor chemical pollutants.* Indoor air contains more toxic chemicals than outdoor air, albeit in smaller concentrations. Chemicals like formaldehyde, benzene, toluene, and xylene are found in common household supplies, office supplies, and building materials. These can cause fatigue, especially in sensitive or allergic patients.

Climatic factors include:

1. *Excess humidity.* Excessive humidity makes it more difficult for the body to cool by perspiration and can lead to fatigue and low energy. Humid climates also harbor more mold and fungi, which can further deplete the sensitive person.

2. *Deficient humidity.* In our cold Minnesota winters, the indoor humidity drops to below 10 percent, drying out mucous membranes and causing sinus congestion, and stuffy noses. In places like the desert southwest, failure to drink adequate fluids in the high heat and low humidity can lead to fatigue.

3. *Deficiency of negative ions.* In certain climates, strong seasonal winds depleted of negative ions blow for weeks. For individuals sensitive to this deficiency of negative ions, the result can be fatigue. For instance, in California a hot, dry, dust-carrying wind known as the Santa Ana blows with great force during winter and spring. This air has a high concentration of positively charged particles and dust, and a low number of negative ions. Some reports have linked these winds to changes in health.

Indoor concentrations of negative ions are almost always too low. This can be remedied by placing a negative ion generator in the room.

4. *Excessive heat.* Prolonged heat exposure can lead to loss of fluids and prolonged release of stress hormones, which may eventually lead to adrenal gland exhaustion. With adrenal exhaustion comes fatigue. Excessive heat exposure may also lead to dehydration, especially if insufficient fluids are consumed or if heavy work is done.

5. *Excess or prolonged cold.* Living in a cold climate can also con-

tribute to fatigue in sensitive individuals. A patient of mine named Judy was ill much of the winter in Minnesota, with fatigue and lethargy being her daily lament. After moving to Arizona her winter doldrums no longer occurred and her general health improved.

6. *Air-conditioned buildings.* According to an article in the *American Journal of Public Health,* air-conditioned buildings "are consistently associated with increased prevalence of work-related headache, lethargy, and upper respiratory/mucous membrane symptoms."[2] If you work in an air-conditioned building, try to notice if your symptoms change when you are in another environment.

In chapter 19, we will discuss a condition called seasonal affective disorder (SAD), which is associated with fatigue and depression and is caused by inadequate sunlight in winter months. Another form of seasonal affective disorder is also being recognized. This form affects people in summer months and is due to high heat and humidity.

Signs and Symptoms

The signs and symptoms that occur due to exposure to airborne substances can affect almost any body system. Headache, rashes, wheezing, infections, fatigue, depression, hyperactivity, earaches, numbness, dizziness, and a host of other symptoms have been reported in people with sensitivity to airborne substances.

Laboratory Tests

There are three categories of tests that might be used to understand your reaction to an airborne substance. The first group includes tests to determine whether you might be reactive to a particular mold, pollen, grass, pollutant, or other substance. The next group includes tests of your environment to determine what types of offenders are present. This is a first step in reducing your exposure. The third category includes tests of your nutrient status, which may give an indication of why you tolerate an airborne substance poorly. For example, if you live in an area with high concentrations of smog it is helpful to know if your antioxidant nutrient status is adequate to protect you.

Tests in the three categories include:

1. Mold plates placed in the bedroom, kitchen, bathroom, and basement, or in your office. These can be obtained from the Northeast Center for Environmental Medicine (2800 W. Genesee St., Syracuse, New York 13219).

2. Intradermal testing for sensitivity to various environmental substances, including mold, pollen, grasses, animals, and chemicals. This is done in the doctor's office.

Blood tests for sensitivity to various environmental substances including mold, pollen, grasses, animals, and chemicals can also be performed. These tests are provided by various laboratories. Serammune Physician's Laboratory in Reston, Virginia, provides the ELISA/ACT test for determining delayed sensitivity to the above categories of substances. Immuno Laboratories in Fort Lauderdale, Florida, also provides tests of environmental substances.

3. Blood tests for nutrient status. See chapter 4.

In Review

1. Airborne substances can cause fatigue in sensitive individuals.

2. Various climatic conditions may also cause fatigue.

3. Testing can help identify whether sensitivity exists.

Chapter 19

Light: Too Little or the Wrong Kind May Make You Tired

LIGHT IS AN ESSENTIAL element of human function. Without the proper amount of light many bodily functions begin to go awry. For example, vitamin D is produced in humans when the skin is exposed to sunlight. This becomes highly seasonally dependent. In one study, people were measured for blood vitamin D content in July, November, and February. In July, blood levels of vitamin D were normal. In November they had declined by 19 percent. By February, vitamin D levels had fallen by 65 percent compared with their July level.[1]

Light also affects mood by virtue of its effect on production of the hormone melatonin, which is highest at nighttime and lowest during the day. Light suppresses secretion of this hormone, while darkness increases its production by the pineal gland (located in the center of the brain). The pineal gland is responsible for orchestrating a number of body rhythms such as day and night cycles, onset of puberty, onset of sleep, and synchronizing our internal clock. The pineal gland is regulated primarily by the kind of light to which we are exposed.

One need only look at plants to see the significance of proper light. If you attempt to grow a plant in the dark, it dies. If you place a plant in a box with a small hole at one end that allows light, the

plant will grow in the direction of the light no matter how convo-
luted it must become in order to achieve this.

The average American spends roughly one hour per day outdoors. The bulk of our time is spent indoors under artificial light.
In most schools, businesses, factories, laboratories, and institutions,
this means fluorescent light. In most homes this means incandescent lights. Both are less than optimum for human functioning, but
fluorescent lights tend to produce more problems.

To understand the differences between the two most common
forms of artificial lighting it is important to understand the nature
of the light we receive from the sun. The sun emits waves of radiant
energy of many types. The light we see is a part of the *visible spectrum* and consists of a composite of the colors red, orange, yellow,
green, blue, indigo, and violet. The different colors are a result of
different wavelengths of light. The length of these waves range between 400 and 700 nanometers. Humans evolved to function under
the complete spectrum of light.

Incandescent lights (like the ones you screw into the lamp socket)
are deficient in the blue end of the spectrum and contain almost no
ultraviolet light. Fluorescent lights come in varying types, but the
most common cool-white fluorescent is deficient in the red and blue-
violet ends of the spectrum. These are precisely the areas in which
the sun's emissions are strongest.[2] Fluorescent lights also emit small
amounts of radiation and have a tendency to flicker slightly, which
can be irritating to one who must spend any amount of time in their
presence.

Inappropriate light, or malillumination, has been linked to the
development of fatigue and low vitality. There are two primary ways
in which this might happen:

- Seasonal deficiency of sunlight in winter months, especially in
  northern climates.
- Prolonged indoor exposure to the incomplete spectrum of fluorescent or incandescent light.

Seasonal Deficiency of Light

In Norway and Finland, decreased exposure to sunlight in winter months correlates with a higher incidence of fatigue, illness, insomnia, depression, irritability, alcoholism, and suicide.[3] In 1981, Dr. Norman Rosenthal described a condition he called seasonal affective disorder (SAD), attributed to decreased sunlight exposure during winter months. For example, SAD was found to affect more than 30 percent of those studied in Nashua, New Hampshire, compared with only 8.9 percent in Sarasota, Florida.[4] It is estimated that approximately 25 million people in the United States suffer from SAD. Many scientists are now in agreement that seasonal affective disorder is a real condition that affects large numbers of people. Those most commonly affected include:[5]

• People living in northern climates.

• Women (4 to 1 over men).

• Adults between the ages of 20 and 40.

A recent study has found that some who suffer from SAD may have underlying thyroid problems.[6] This may be worth investigating if you suffer from SAD.

Signs of SAD commonly include: Depressed mood, decreased concentration, interpersonal problems, mood swings, fatigue, reduced sex drive, irritability, and other symptoms common to depression often occur in SAD. However, additional symptoms occur with SAD that are not common with other forms of depression. They include:

| Increased sleep | Increased appetite |
| Weight gain | Carbohydrate craving |

Numerous clinics around the country now use a widely accepted treatment to care for patients with SAD—daily exposure to bright, full-spectrum light. According to Michael Hill, M.D., director of the Seasonal Disorders Clinic at the University of North Carolina School of Medicine, no study using bright light to treat SAD has failed to find a significant positive effect on symptoms.[7]

Many different parameters such as brightness, color, duration, distance, and spectrum are important in determining the outcome of light treatment. The most common treatment today is done with full-spectrum fluorescent light at 10,000 Lux for 30 minutes each morning.[8]

If you suffer from seasonal depression and suspect it may be due to SAD, don't simply rely on light therapy until you've ruled out other causes of depression. Also, if you seem to suffer from SAD, but also have an eye disorder such as macular degeneration, *do not embark on any form of light therapy until your doctors have made a full evaluation.* Viewing bright light can cause further damage in some eye disorders.

Melatonin is being used by some doctors to treat SAD. Recall that melatonin is a hormone produced by the pineal gland. It is produced in greatest amounts during darkness and least in light. We will probably hear much more about this treatment of SAD in the coming years.

Fluorescent Light

Exposure to fluorescent light that is not full-spectrum presents another problem. Many people spend eight to ten hours a day under fluorescent lights. Some individuals don't seem to be particularly bothered by them, but others find that fluorescent lights make them irritable, fatigued, and less productive. In some people, fluorescent lights also trigger headaches. Mark, a former patient of mine studying to be a doctor, was so sensitive to fluorescent lights that he would nearly fall asleep reading x-rays. This did not bode well for his final examination in radiology. To study for the test he had to sit and look at x-rays on a viewbox (with fluorescent lights as the light source) for hours at a time. While some of the students were able to view x-rays for several hours, he found he could only spend about 30 minutes at a time before needing a break. He took his exams and passed with flying colors, but to this day he becomes fatigued if he spends too much time under fluorescent lights.

Jeffrey was an 11-year-old boy who became fatigued toward the middle of the school day. As his fatigue set in he found he could only remain alert by rocking in his seat. This created quite a stir among his classmates and especially irritated the teacher. He was fine at home, but by mid-afternoon at school the same pattern emerged. He had seen many doctors, the school counselor, and, of course, the principal.

Through a series of blinded tests I conducted in my office, it became clear that Jeffrey was very sensitive to the fluorescent lights in his classroom. I suggested one of two options: that they move Jeffrey's chair near the window and turn off that bank of lights, or they leave him in his present location and turn off all the fluorescent lights in the room. The teacher, somewhat skeptical, agreed to keep the lights off except for those over her desk for one week. Jeffrey and the teacher were both happy with the results. However, she did not see a darkened room for the remainder of the school year as a reasonable compromise. They agreed to move his desk near the window and turn off one bank of lights.

If you work under fluorescent lights and have some control over the situation you may wish to either turn them off and work in a poorly illumined room, turn them off and add a lamp to the room, or replace fluorescents with full-spectrum fluorescents. I once treated stockbroker with chronic fatigue and chemical sensitivity who was also highly sensitive to fluorescent lights. He occupied a corner office on the 40th floor of the IDS Tower in downtown Minneapolis with a spectacular view of the city. He found that keeping the fluorescent lights off improved his energy.

In Review

1. Light is important in helping to regulate various body functions.

2. Many people receive inadequate sunlight exposure, especially in northern climates.

3. Insufficient sunlight in winter months leads to a form of

depression and fatigue called seasonal affective disorder (SAD) in susceptible people.

4. Light therapy is the treatment of choice for SAD.

5. Fluorescent lights may produce fatigue in sensitive individuals.

6. Try to get more sunlight on sunny days during winter months.

Chapter 20

Sleep and Rest

ACCORDING TO THE Institute of Medicine, roughly one-third of Americans experience some form of sleep difficulty. Data complied by the American Sleep Disorders Association reveals that accidents and loss of productivity due to sleep deprivation cost Americans $50 billion per year. Fatigue and low vitality are among the first consequences of sleep deprivation. If you are frequently or constantly tired, you should evaluate the amount of sleep and rest you get each day. Individual sleep needs vary from person to person. The range is from six to ten hours a day. According to Sanford Auerback, M.D., director of the Sleep Disorders Center at Boston University, people in general do not get as much sleep as they need to function optimally. He adds, "We are a very sleep-deprived society."[1]

Your sleep cycles depend on a balance of brain chemicals known as neurotransmitters. The main chemicals include serotonin and glycine, the so-called sleep-promoting compounds, and epinephrine, norepinephrine, and dopamine. The latter three are stimulating and promote wakefulness. Diet, nutrition, and exercise play a very important role in the balance of these chemicals. When the activity of serotonin and glycine prevail in the brain, you become sleepy. When the activity of epinephrine (adrenalin) and dopamine predominate, you become alert and energized.

One means of promoting restful sleep is to encourage the production of the proper neurotransmitters at the appropriate time of day. This can be done with diet, nutritional supplements, exercise, and with deep abdominal breathing techniques.

Devon is an example of how poor sleep may contribute to fatigue. At age 39, he always felt tired and fell asleep often during the day. Reading a book was difficult because he could not stay awake, even during daytime hours. He sometimes fell asleep during conversations and needed daytime naps. To cope, he drank large amounts of coffee. An analysis of his behavior during sleep was highly revealing. During deep sleep, he stopped breathing for extended periods (sleep apnea). At one point, his breathing stopped for one minute twenty seconds. When his breathing stopped, the oxygen saturation of his blood dropped dramatically. While roughly 98 percent saturation is normal, Devon's levels fell to as low as 70 percent. The episodes during which he stopped breathing were not isolated, but were quite regular throughout the night—up to 50 times an hour. With such disrupted sleep and such low oxygen saturation, it is not surprising that he was tired all the time.

His therapy has been to sleep with a device (called a CPAP), that ensures air flow into the nose so that breathing is maintained at a constant level during sleep. Using this apparatus, his oxygen saturation is kept above 90 percent. After only 48 hours use, Devon noticed substantial improvement in energy. Eight weeks later, he described his energy as dramatically improved. He can now go with less sleep and still function well.

Poor sleep, inadequate sleep, or insomnia can be a result of many different factors. As you review this list, keep in mind that insomnia is also associated with various medical conditions. You should see your doctor to rule these out. Common factors that contribute to poor sleep are listed below.

Diet. A number of foods, food allergens, and food additives can contribute to poor sleep. These include caffeinated beverages such as coffee and cola. Also included are individual foods to which you may be intolerant. A 32-year-old patient of mine had to wake three to four times each night to urinate and found it difficult to get back to sleep after each trip to the bathroom. She was fatigued through-out the day as a result of her interrupted and inadequate sleep. We later found that she had an allergy to cow's milk. Once the cow's milk was removed from her diet, she no longer awoke at night and her sleep improved.

Illness. There are numerous medical conditions associated with insomnia or poor sleep. Examples include urinary disorders, thyroid dysfunction, nasal and sinus problems, reflux esophagitis and hiatal hernia, anxiety disorders, depression, asthma, gallbladder disease, and others. Chronic pain may also interfere with sleep.

Medication. There is a wide range of drugs that interfere with sleep. Included are asthma medication, sleeping pills, hormones, antihypertensives, and many others. Moreover, certain drugs given to *induce* sleep, i.e., sleeping pills, may also cause chronic fatigue. For example, Halcyon and Restoril have a high capacity to induce fatigue. Tranquilizers such as Librium, Mellaril, and others like them cause symptoms of chronic fatigue as well.[2] If you have difficulty sleeping and are on medication, look up your medication in the *Physicians' Desk Reference* at the library and then see your doctor about a possible change. Don't just stop your medication without consulting your doctor.

Television. Late-night TV viewing can lead to poor sleep, especially if news, violence, or action-oriented shows are viewed.

Parenting. If you are a parent of a small child you probably spell SLEEP DEPRIVATION with capital letters. I know I did with my two boys. This is a most difficult time that eventually passes. However, while in the midst of it you want to develop coping skills.

Exercise. If you don't get adequate physical activity, chances are your sleep will not be as sound. Beginning an exercise program (often as simple as walking) may be what you need. Make sure you don't start out too vigorously. Begin gently, increase gradually, but keep increasing your level of activity.

Those who exercise regularly may also have sleep difficulty. The two prime culprits are exercising in the evening before bed, which creates an arousal state, and overtraining. Athletes who overtrain frequently experience insomnia. In fact, insomnia is one of the key diagnostic points to consider when assessing whether the overtraining syndrome exists.

Shift Work. A large number of people work night shifts or rotating shifts that interfere with normal sleep rhythms. In one study, 56 percent of night shift workers reported falling asleep on the job.[3] For those on rotating shifts a possible solution has been found at the Sleep-Wake Disorders Center in White Plains, New York. They found that exposing workers to extra-bright lights for the first four hours on the first overnight shift adjusts workers' clocks to the new schedule almost instantly. Interestingly, shift workers who truly love their work seem to have less sleep difficulty than those who dislike their work. Another solution being studied is administration of melatonin, a sleep-inducing hormone produced by the body at night.

Sleep Apnea. Sleep apnea is a condition in which breathing is interrupted during sleep. This results in inadequate distribution of oxygen to the tissues. There are two kinds of sleep apnea: obstructive and central. Obstructive sleep apnea usually occurs in those who snore. These individuals wake frequently during the night due to cessation of breathing, which partially accounts for their fatigue during the day. If you are chronically tired and are told by a friend or spouse that you snore, there is a good chance you suffer from obstructive sleep apnea. Central sleep apnea is less common and is due to a problem with the brain signaling the respiratory muscles to breathe. Snoring is not a typical symptom with this form of apnea.

Some cases of sleep apnea may be related to chemical exposure. Sixty-six men exposed to solvents on the job were assessed for sleep apnea. Sleep apnea occurred in roughly one-fifth of the men (compared with about 1 in 100 in the general population), which prompted the investigators to conclude that some cases of sleep apnea may be solvent-induced encephalopathy.[4]

Anxiety/Depression. Anxiety or depression can lead to poor sleep. Fatigue then leads to exhaustion, which can aggravate the anxiety or depressive state. Exercise is often helpful in alleviating anxiety and can improve depressive states in many people. The underlying cause of the disorders should be sought.

Light. Inadequate or improper light exposure can contribute to sleep difficulty. Lack of adequate sunlight in winter months can contribute to SAD, a form of depression that is characterized by poor sleep and fatigue. Full-spectrum light treatment is often indicated, and patients are also urged to spend time outdoors with at least their face and hands exposed to the sun. Exposure to fluorescent lights in the workplace can also cause irritability that adversely influences sleep.

Nutritional Deficiency. Deficiency of nutrients may alter sleep patterns. Magnesium deficiency is known to trigger insomnia. In one study, 99 percent of 200 people with insomnia improved after starting a magnesium supplement.[5] Copper deficiency or excess may cause insomnia. Patients with low iron intake may have difficulty sleeping, but remember, iron supplements should not be taken unless blood tests have shown you are deficient.

Deficiency of the amino acid tryptophan can lead to diminished serotonin production and poor sleep. Vitamin B_6 is needed to convert tryptophan to serotonin, so deficiency of B_6 may also lead to sleep difficulty. In fact, giving vitamin B_6 increases dream, or REM, sleep in some people. Niacin also seems to increase REM sleep. Some people who take tryptophan for sleep find that they fall asleep easily, but wake in the night. According to Eric Braverman, M.D., these patients often require more tryptophan than they had been given, or additional B_6 or niacin.[6]

Chemical Exposure. In 112 individuals evaluated for exposure to organic solvents (house paints, spray finishers, printing), there was a significantly higher prevalence of insomnia than in those not exposed to solvents.[7] In *Environmental Neurotoxicology,* it is reported that any one of 119 different chemicals can cause sleep disturbance.[8] Chemical exposure may induce sleep disturbances by altering the way in which excitatory and inhibitory neurotransmitters are produced in the brain. Solvent chemicals such as toluene, benzene, trichloroethylene, and others may trigger free-radical reactions once inside the body. Free radicals can trigger the release of adrenalin, the powerful alerting chemical.

Volatile chemicals are present in the homes and workplaces of millions of Americans. If you suffer from poor sleep, evaluate your situation to see if chemical exposure might be part of the problem. When chemical exposure has occurred, nutrient status becomes altered. Thus, it is important that your nutritional status be evaluated.

Signs and Symptoms

> Difficulty falling asleep
> Awakening alert in the middle of the night
> Awakening feeling sluggish in the morning
> Waking frequently in the night

Laboratory Tests

Sleep disorder clinics may run a variety of psychological and neurological tests in an attempt to pinpoint the origins of your sleep difficulty. An assessment of brainwave activity, blood oxygen saturation, breathing rate, and other tests are among these. Standard laboratory tests may be used to rule out medical conditions. A salivary test for cortisol and DHEA may reveal adrenal gland dysfunction, which can contribute to altered sleep. Nutritional assessment may indicate nutrient abnormalities that interfere with sleep. Tests for food intolerance may also be revealing.

Natural Remedies

If you have trouble sleeping you may wish to try 400 to 500 mg of magnesium glycinate or magnesium citrate. Recall the study in which 99 percent of 200 people with insomnia improved after starting a magnesium supplement.[9] In one study of valerian root and insomnia, 44 percent reported perfect sleep and 89 percent reported improved sleep with no side effects.[10]

Essential (plant) oils: Basil, camphor, chamomile, lavender, marjoram,* neroli,* rose, sandalwood, and ylang-ylang have all been shown to improve insomnia.[11] Robert Tisserand recommends mixing 12 drops bergamot, 4 drops geranium, and 9 drops sandalwood into 50 mls of vegetable oil. This can be massaged onto the shoulders or back before bed to promote a relaxed, restful sleep. (Note: avoid sun exposure when bergamot is used on the skin.) Kurt

Schnaubelt, Ph.D., of San Rafael, California, has used heliotrope to aid in sleep.[12]

Avoid caffeine consumption via coffee, tea, or soda pop.

One means to achieve better sleep is to practice deep-breathing relaxation exercises every day and before bed. It can aid in reducing the excitatory adrenal hormones and promote formation of the calming serotonergic chemicals in the brain.

Some doctors have begun to use the hormone melatonin in people with sleep disorders. This may prove to be a valuable treatment in the future.

In Review

1. Inadequate sleep and rest are common causes of fatigue.

2. Certain dietary habits and nutritional deficiencies may contribute to poor sleep.

3. Inadequate exercise contributes to poor sleep.

4. Other factors that contribute to poor sleep include chemical exposure, stimulants such as caffeine, prescription drugs, inadequate light, sleep apnea, anxiety or depression, shift work, and a number of medical conditions.

5. Improving quality of sleep improves immune function and reduces fatigue.

Chapter 21

Circumstantial Fatigue

By now it is probably obvious that there is no shortage of physical, chemical, biological, or emotional factors that contribute to fatigue. One factor that you may not have given consideration is that of circumstances. This may ultimately boil down to how you perceive the circumstances, how you act upon them, and what you do to change your situation. However, there is no doubt that our circumstances can take quite a toll on us.

Work seems to be one of the most common and difficult forms of circumstantial fatigue. If you feel stuck with an irate, nasty boss, life can be pretty difficult. Alternately, you might thoroughly enjoy your work, but a co-worker with whom you must closely associate is a nag, a bore, and a gossip. Being without a job can be stressful as well.

Family situations may also produce enormous fatigue. In many cases, the body or mind literally shuts down or goes to sleep in an effort to avoid the pain of the circumstance. This happened when Marion's father ended up in a nursing home, while at the same time her mother grew more feeble and less able to care for herself. Marion felt as though she spent all of her free moments visiting her father, running errands and chauffeuring her mother, and attending to their financial matters. What was perhaps most difficult was the constant complaining Marion had to endure from her father. Marion felt tired and sleepy almost all the time. Her performance at work suffered.

Her marriage suffered. Her relationship with her married children suffered. Her happiness suffered.

Marion suffered from a variety of physical ailments, which were not serious, merely constant. She spent a lot of money and time trying to remedy her physical symptoms. I pointed out that she had to take control of the situation regarding her family or her physical symptoms and fatigue would probably continue.

One suggestion was to speak up to her father rather than simply endure his insults and bickering. The thought of this frightened her, but at the same time gave her sense of power and relief. She received a boost of energy just visualizing herself saying, "Dad, I'm not going to take your endless criticism. Either you quit complaining, quit degrading me, and treat me with respect, or you can find someone else to take care of you."

Living in an abusive relationship is form of situational fatigue that drains enormous amounts of energy and contributes to chronic illness. This is a tragic circumstance that is not so easily remedied. It is essential that emotional and physical support be found that will help alter the situation. If emotional, sexual, or physical abuse has taken place in the past, it is important to seek some form of counseling. Researchers at the University of Medicine and Dentistry of New Jersey assessed the effects of childhood abuse on the rate of illness in women. Fifty-three percent of the women reported suffering one or more kinds of abuse (physical, emotional, or sexual) as children. The women reporting abuse were more likely to report symptoms of fatigue, insomnia, and headaches.[1]

Clutter presents another situation that can contribute to fatigue. I define clutter as unnecessary or unfinished things that persist and occupy our attention. We can have emotional clutter or physical clutter. Emotional clutter might include letters we haven't written, phone calls we haven't made, a stack of "things to do" notes lying around the house, plans for the family vacation, an unresolved argument in which we no longer speak to the person, failure to assert ourselves in a relationship, unresolved issues between you and your parents/spouse/children, and so on. Each of us has a long list of unfinished items that occupy our minds, cluttering up our thoughts. You will almost always find that clearing away the clutter from your mind gives you a needed boost of energy.

Physical clutter is another form of clutter that can drain your batteries. If your house, desk, office, or car is a mess with things lying all around, the clutter can be a negative force. Our house was filled with far too many toys that had been given to our oldest son. The house was likewise filled with items that *we* no longer used or needed—they were just lying around gathering dust. We decided to clear out our spaces and give our unused things to needy children. The feeling after freeing ourselves of all this "stuff" was invigorating.

Another form of mental/emotional clutter is over-commitment. Any parent knows that you can become worn out by hauling your children to different functions every night of the week. Add to this your own commitments to church, civic groups, friends, work, school, or whatever else and the effect can be substantial. The key here is to prioritize. What do you really need to do and what could you do without? Sit in a relaxed state and then image your commitments one by one. How would you feel if you dropped one or more of them? Would it help to simplify your life?

Stressful life events can also produce circumstantial fatigue. The death of a family member, loss of a job, beginning a new relationship, moving to a new city, deadlines at work, and many other events can lower your energy. When Holmes and Rahe developed their Social Readjustment Rating Scale, they discovered that people who scored above 300 points were far more likely to be hospitalized within the next year than those with lower scores. The scale was a measure of life events. The more stressful events occurring at one time, the greater the score. Stress and life events are also known to bring about declines in immune function. In *Beyond Antibiotics*, a lengthy chapter is devoted to the effects of mood, mind, and stress on immune function.

Some people feel fatigued by their circumstances because they feel unsupported, that they are bearing the burden alone. One of your actions might be to confide in someone about your dilemma. Another might be to ask for help from a friend, sibling, or co-worker. Often the frustration arises because you have asked for help and no one is willing or able to come to your aid. Perhaps you need to hire someone to help in other aspects of your life.

What you must do in all situations that produce difficulty for you is *take action*. Doing nothing almost always ensures that the problem will not go away and that it will likely get worse. The action can take almost any form that seems appropriate to you, as long as your action either changes the situation or you change the way you relate to or perceive the situation.

Tests for Circumstantial Fatigue

There are obviously no laboratory tests to help determine whether you suffer from circumstantial or situational fatigue. You will want to look carefully at the times when you are fatigued and see whether it may be related to your present circumstances.

Make a list of the five most difficult circumstances with which you are faced. Next, write a brief note about how each situation makes you feel. Then make a list of how you might change each situation so that it does not impact your wellbeing so significantly. I'll give you a clue—in every instance you will want to change your perception of the situation. You will then want to list specific actions that you can take to change the situations themselves.

Wally is a good example. He felt so tired every afternoon that he "just had to take a nap." These were not your average twenty-minute siestas, but full-fledged, two-hour, mid-afternoon sojourns. Wally owned his own business writing computer software and worked out of his home. He spent a lot of time working alone and was not pleased with the progress his business was making. His solution was to escape it all by sleeping away a large part of the business day. We discussed a better solution. First, he needed to find ways to increase his contact with other people, especially people with similar business interests. Second, he needed to look carefully at his business and see why it was not performing well. It turned out that Wally was a gifted programmer, but he spent very little time and energy on marketing.

Wally took active steps to increase his professional interaction. He also invited a consultant to see how to best market his skills and products. His energy began to change almost immediately after he began making changes. As his business improved, not only did he not sleep each afternoon, but he found himself working late into the evening on occasion.

Not all cases work out so well and not all circumstances are so easily changed. Moreover, some people are so resistant to change that they sabotage their own recovery efforts. As I said, doing nothing is the best way to ensure that your circumstantial fatigue will remain unchanged. What the above success stories have in common is that each person was committed to changing and took specific action.

According to Richard Podell, M.D., author of *Doctor, Why Am I So Tired?*, the litmus test for determining if your fatigue is situational or circumstantial is to note the feelings you are having about your present situation and then sense your reaction to a more pleasant prospect. If there is a significant improvement in your energy, chances are your fatigue is circumstantial. Often the excitement of something you want to do erases the fatigue.[2] If you want to see this in action, try it out on your children. I asked my son to clean up his room. "Dad, I'm too tired" was his retort. He actually had had a long day and was pretty tired. I then said, "How would you like to go to the Timberwolves game against the Chicago Bulls tonight?" He instantly changed his state, jumped out of the chair, and said, "That would be great, Dad!" His fatigue was clearly circumstantial.

In Review

1. Circumstances can cause one to feel fatigued.

2. Often it is our perception of the circumstances that causes an adverse reaction in our bodies.

3. One way to assess whether your fatigue is circumstantial is to note the feelings you are having about your present situation and then sense your reaction to a more pleasant prospect. If there is a significant improvement in your energy, chances are your fatigue is circumstantial.

4. Improving fatigue that is circumstantial usually involves changing your perception and taking action.

Chapter 22

Psychological Factors and Fatigue: Depression, Stress, Beliefs, and Optimism

SOME OF THE most exciting scientific research of this century surrounds the Western discovery of the link between mind and body. The ancient Chinese, the ancient Egyptians, and Native people from around the globe have known of this link for centuries. Yet, the explosion of knowledge that now verifies these time-honored observations gives us great understanding, hope, and inspiration as we grapple with modern diseases.

Chronic fatigue is, as we've seen, a vague disorder with myriad causes. The mind/body link in chronic fatigue is as important as any known physical cause. Indeed, in almost all cases of chronic fatigue there is some psychological factor at work. The difficulty is knowing which comes first, the fatigue or the emotional state. Far too many people have been told by a doctor, unable to find a physical cause for the symptoms, that it is all in their head. The person is labeled a psychiatric case and sent off for counseling. Counseling may indeed be helpful, but this manner of dealing with the situation trivializes the importance and complexity of the emotional state. Moreover, it separates the doctor from treatment of the whole person. Instead of having a doctor who will work closely with you on all aspects of your care, you have one doctor who can't find anything physically wrong and one who thinks it is all in your mind. The truth of the matter is that in almost *all* cases of illness, the mind and the body are both involved.

If you suffer from fatigue, low vitality, and tiredness you must understand that there *is definitely* a psychological component to your condition. This is nothing of which to be ashamed. It is only a reflection of the natural way in which our bodies' were designed to function. Our moods and emotional states have a profound effect on our physiology, our immune systems, our digestive enzymes, and on virtually all aspects of bodily function. Our physical state of being has a significant impact on our emotional state. In essence, the mind is connected to *everything* that happens in the body at every moment.

We could discuss many different psychological factors relative to fatigue. However, depression, stress, beliefs, and optimism seem to be particularly relevant and are the ones I will discuss here.

Depression

Depression is among the most common emotional illnesses, affecting an estimated 11 million people in the U.S. every six months. One in five Americans will experience depression at some point in their lifetime. Women are twice as likely as men to be affected by depression. Everybody feels sadness, dejection, and changes in mood. However, depression is long-lasting and often recurrent.

There are different forms of depression as well as different causes. Some of the most common factors that contribute to depression are discussed below.

Nutritional Status. Nutritional status can affect mood so profoundly that depression may result. Melvyn Werbach, M.D., clinical professor of medicine at the University of California at Los Angeles, is author of a book entitled *Nutritional Influences on Mental Illness.* In his book he reviews hundreds of studies relative to the effect specific nutrient deficiencies may have on development of depression. The most common nutrients cited in his book are: biotin, folic acid, pyridoxine, riboflavin, thiamin, vitamin B12, vitamin C, calcium, copper, iron, magnesium, and potassium. He also discusses several nutritional substances that have antidepressive properties. These include lithium, phenylalanine, tyrosine, tryptophan, S-adenosyl-L-methionine, and hypericin.[1]

Psychiatrist Priscilla Slagle, in her book *The Way Up from Down,* discusses nutritional causes and therapies for depression. It is her contention that the majority of cases of depression result in biochemical dysregulation. Vitamins, minerals, and amino acids are the bricks and mortar of brain neurochemicals. If we can identify where deficiencies and biochemical blocks exist, we can tailor a nutrition program to enhance brain function. Slagle's book is filled with many case studies and a discussion of nutrients used in managing depression. Using a method called precursor loading, she has been able to restore normal function to patients suffering from depression.[2] Precursor loading describes a practice wherein the raw nutrients needed to form a certain neurotransmitter are given to enhance the production of that neurotransmitter.

She is hardly alone among those who advocate a nutritional/biochemical model for depression and other psychiatric illness. Scientists at the National Insitutes of Health recently convened a conference on the role of omega-3 fatty acids in psychiatric disease. This work is based on the fact that the human brain is roughly sixty percent fat and that fatty acids have a profound affect upon brain structure and function. In fact, there are now over fifty disorders of the brain that may related to fatty acid imbalance. Fatty acids are increasingly seen as an important nutritional factor in depression. (See *Smart Fats: How Dietary Fats and Oils Affect Mental, Physical, and Emotional Intelligence,* Schmidt, MA. North Atlantic Books.)

A study conducted by Aatron Medical Laboratories illustrates the importance of assessing nutrient levels in mood disorders. In a study of more than 500 people, none had normal blood amino acid levels. Low tyrosine, phenylalanine, and tryptophan were common. Half of the subjects had low glutamine.[4]

Another interesting relationship with dietary and nutritional correlates is blood histamine. Dr. Carl Pfeiffer noted many years ago that blood histamine had a profound effect on mood. He noted that people with either high or low blood histamine had very characteristic forms of depression. Blood histamine levels and mood could be managed in these people by specific nutrient protocols and dietary modifications.[5] Histamine levels can be measured in blood.

Treatment protocols for the high and low histamine types are available from doctors who work with orthomolecular psychiatry or clinical nutrition.

Food Intolerance. Food intolerance may also bring on symptoms of depression, which can then lead to fatigue. One such case was Carolyn. She had been depressed for about four years. The onset of her depression was initially unexplained. As we reviewed her history it seemed that her depression began about the time she had been treated for a nasty bladder infection. She had been given antibiotics in large doses for the initial infection, but recurrences were common so heavier, more frequent doses were subsequently used. Her bladder infection was finally brought under control. However, her mood began to deteriorate. Depression followed.

Looking at her diet history it was clear that she craved wheat and dairy products—a connection she had not previously made. I had her begin an elimination diet wherein she would eat no wheat or dairy products for six weeks. Her mood steadily improved. She described it as "a cloud clearing overhead to reveal a sunny blue sky."

Next came the true test. Would her depressive symptoms return if she ate wheat or dairy products again? This could only be learned from a challenge with the offending foods. I instructed her to drink a glass of milk in the clinic. We would observe any adverse reactions and deal with any crisis that might follow. She drank four ounces of milk and was quickly overcome with feelings of sleepiness, fatigue, irritability, and headache. This quickly degenerated into crying, fogginess, inability to concentrate, and outbursts of anger. In a few hours, her symptoms of depression returned. She felt hopeless, helpless, and depressed. It was a rather dramatic shift from her mood prior to the challenge. Carolyn was able to get over her depression by avoiding wheat- and dairy-containing foods.

Not all cases of depression are so simple and many do not have a significant allergic component. However, food allergy and intolerance exert such a profound effect on mood that they should always be considered whenever depression exists. One study found 33 percent of depressed patients had allergies compared to only 2 percent of a group of schizophrenics.[6] A study of 30 patients complaining of depression, confusion, and other symptoms showed reactivity to multiple allergens, which worsened their behavioral symptoms.[7]

Circumstantial. Depression can also occur as a result of difficult circumstances such as impending divorce, death of a child or a spouse, legal troubles, IRS audits, and a lengthy list of other factors. Emotional, physical, or sexual abuse can also bring about depression. This can occur if the abuse is ongoing or if it has happened in the distant past. If you suffer from depression as a result of circumstances such as these, it is important that you have the support of family and loved ones and that you develop healthy coping skills. In many such cases professional counseling is very important, especially if you have any desire to harm yourself.

Chronic Illness. Depression is common in people with chronic illness. The difficulty of living with chronic pain, chronic disability, or impaired function is often a trigger of depression. Chronic illness can strain relationships. It can cause one to lose a job, which may deal a further blow to self-esteem and self-worth. The lack of physical activity that goes with chronic illness can itself contribute to depression and fatigue. In many people with chronic fatigue, depression is not so much a cause of fatigue as it is a result of being constantly tired and unable to perform normal daily duties.

Thyroid Dysfunction. Depression can be a symptom of poor thyroid function. In a group of 16 patients with depression, 56 percent had subclinical hypothyroidism.[8]

Adrenal Insufficiency. Adrenal insufficiency can be a cause of biological depression. This occurs when important adrenal steroid hormones such as cortisol and DHEA (dehydroepiandrosterone) are not produced in proper amounts or are not well regulated at certain times of day. In fact, elevated cortisol at midnight indicates a form of depression known as endogenous depression. This can be helped enormously by restoring adrenal gland balance. Adrenal insufficiency is often triggered by various stressors such as physical, chemical, or emotional trauma. Chronic stress such as that commonly encountered in Western society is also a contributor to poor adrenal function. In a study of people with adrenal insufficiency, depression was reported in 79 percent.[9]

Chemical Exposure. The brain and nervous system are among the first targets of chemical exposure. This is because the brain and nervous system are made primarily of fat. Most of the chemical solvents, pesticides, herbicides, and other pollutants are fat-soluble, meaning they have an especially high affinity for the delicate tissues of the nervous system. Symptoms of depression, lethargy, fatigue, confusion, poor memory, and others are common following chemical exposure. This is especially the case in people who are chemically sensitive.

Inadequate Sunlight. Inadequate sunlight in the winter months can lead to a form of depression known as Seasonal Affective Disorder (SAD). Some cases of SAD may also be associated with sluggish thyroid function. This is discussed in greater depth in chapter 19.

View of Self. How one views oneself can be the origin of depression in many, many cases. This can be related to experiences that occurred in childhood that have influenced a person's sense of self-worth.

Genetics. There is some genetic basis for depression. However, even these cases may be influenced by nutritional and metabolic intervention.

Signs and Symptoms

Self-criticism	Sense of failure
Suicidal feelings	Sense of punishment
Loss of social interest	Sadness
Uninterested in life	Lack of purpose
Moodiness	Unmotivated
Insomnia	Tiredness, fatigue
Loss of sex drive	Excessive crying
Lack of energy	Eating too much or too little

Laboratory Tests

Various tests in the field of functional medicine might be used to determine if your depression is due to a nutritional, endocrine, or metabolic imbalance. These may include but are not limited to the following:

- Thyroid function tests
- Neurotransmitters such as epinephrine, serotonin, etc. (24-hour urine)
- Salivary cortisol. Measured at 8 A.M., 12 P.M., 4 P.M., and 11 P.M.
- Salivary DHEA (dehydroepiandrosterone)
- Whole blood histamine
- IgE or IgG tests for food sensitivity. IgG is a better test for delayed reactions.
- Tests for vitamin and mineral status
- Urine or plasma amino acids
- Urine organic acid analysis

There are various personality inventories, such as the Beck Depression Index, that can be taken to determine if depression exists. A thorough history is also important.

Treatment

Physicians still rely heavily on antidepressive medication to treat depression in their patients. Some people are helped by the medication while others are not. If you are in a crisis situation, medication may be extremely helpful to get you through the crisis.

Some doctors believe that tricyclic antidepressants are effective because they are potent antihistamines. If depression is due to allergy or high histamine (at least some cases), then it makes sense that these potent antihistamines would improve symptoms of depression.[10]

There are two important factors regarding antidepressants. While sometimes helpful, these drugs do not address the cause of the depression. If it is nutritional, metabolic, related to allergy, related to chemical exposure, related to beliefs or attitudes, or many other possible factors, the drug will deal primarily with symptoms. The underlying cause should still be sought.

Second, antidepressant drugs sometimes *produce* fatigue as a pri-

mary side effect. Elavil, Sinequan, Desyrel, and others all have extremely high capacity to induce fatigue. On a scale of zero to three,
with three being the highest fatigue-inducing potential, Podell rates
these drugs a three.[11] Thus, if you suffer from chronic fatigue you
do not want to be taking a drug that produces fatigue as a major side
effect.

Two of the most popular antidepressants in the United States are
Prozac and Zoloft. Prozac (fluoxetine) and Zoloft (sertraline) are in
a family of drugs known as selective serotonin reuptake inhibitors
(SSRI). These drugs can be very helpful in certain cases of depression and chronic fatigue. In the case of Dr. Tom, which I'll describe
later, Zoloft made a substantial difference in his mood. He felt that
he could function more easily and was relatively free of depressive
symptoms. However, he also recognized that it was not getting at
the cause of his problem. This represents one of the fundamental
concerns about such drugs. It is believed that many doctors are prescribing them without a thorough psychological evaluation. In lib-
erally prescribing these antidepressants, doctors may be overlooking
important psychological aspects for which counseling might be more
appropriate. They may also overlook physical findings suggestive of
an organic or biochemical cause that would go untreated if Prozac
or Zoloft were relied upon as the primary treatment.[12]

Certain drugs given to induce sleep (i.e., sleeping pills) may also
cause chronic fatigue. For example, Halcion and Restoril have a high
capacity to induce fatigue. Tranquilizers such as Librium, Mellaril,
and others like them cause symptoms of chronic fatigue as well. If
you are on any of these medications, consult your doctor to see if
the drug might be a part of your fatigue problem and if you might
look more deeply for the origins of your depression.[13]

If you are depressed, you and your doctor should investigate the
following possibilities and take the appropriate therapeutic action:

Allergies	Nutritional deficiency
Hypothyroidism	Chemical exposure
Belief system	Life events
Circumstances	Blood sugar abnormality

Lack of physical activity   Disease state
Prescription drugs   Alcohol, illicit drugs
Core psychological issues

Given the growing evidence that mood disorders such as depression reflect an imbalance in neurotransmitters that can be improved with nutrition, it seems only logical that nutritional status be carefully assessed in all cases.

Stress

Stress is a natural part of each of our lives. If we lived without stress there would be little to challenge and stimulate us. Yet it is obvious that if we live under constant stress we may become overwhelmed and succumb to disease. Many studies have shown the effect of stress on development of illness. The immune system is acutely responsive to stress. In studies of children, stress was related to the duration and severity of illness.[14] In a Harvard study of families, those under high stress who tested positive for the strep bacteria were almost three times more likely to get sick than those under low stress who were also culture-positive for strep.[15] In studies of five common cold viruses, those under stress were much more likely to become infected when exposed and to develop a cold after exposure.[16]

All of these studies show the effects of stress on the immune system, which is important when talking about chronic fatigue. However, in each study there were people under stress who did not get sick. This same phenomenon occurs in real life. What is the secret? The secret appears to be related, in part, to attitude and coping. Those who have good skills for coping with stress do not seem to be affected to nearly the same degree as those with poor coping skills.

Different responses of the so-called Type A and Type B personalities is a good example of the varied response to stress. People who are Type A tend to be extremely competitive, aggressive, hasty, impatient, achievement-oriented, and time-urgent. Type A people produce more stress hormones and free fatty acids after stress than Type B people. When Type A people are challenged by stress, they release more magnesium from their blood cells and eliminate more of this vital nutrient through the urine. In an article published in the *Journal of the American College of Nutrition*, 80 percent of Type A people exposed to stress experienced a drop in red cell magnesium, while only 44 percent of Type B people experienced this decline.[17]

In one who is constantly stressed, this periodic loss of magnesium might lead to significant magnesium deficiency. Not only does this put the heart at risk, since heart muscle needs magnesium to function properly, but it may lead to significant fatigability in general. Recall the earlier chapter on vitamins and minerals where it was noted that magnesium deficiency was a common finding in fatigued patients regardless of their overall state of health. Also recall the words of Dr. Stephen Davies, who said, "CFS patients are almost always deficient in magnesium."[18]

A lengthy discussion of stress is not possible here, but please recognize that stress and one's ability to cope can have a profound effect on energy.

Beliefs

Many years ago, there were three men who walked down a path in India at different times of day. The first man sauntered joyfully down the path when suddenly he was startled by the presence of a large cobra. He was struck with terror. His heart pounded wildly. His instinct was to run, but he could not. Certain he would be struck and killed, he was paralyzed by fear—traumatized by the threat to his life. The second man was a herpetologist, one who studies snakes. He walked down this same path, stumbled upon the snake, but was struck with fascination at this large, graceful creature. He gazed at the snake with keen interest, studying its every movement, observing the flare of its head, the pulsation of its breathing, the deep stare of its eyes, the texture of its skin. He was thrilled by the opportunity to see this magnificent creature in the wild. The third man—a Hindu holy man—walked down the path, stumbled upon the snake, and fell to his knees in prayer. To the Hindu, the cobra is revered. The holy man was struck with awe, humility, and gratitude to be in the presence of this creature.

Each man came face to face with a deadly animal. Yet their responses to the encounter were radically different, based upon their beliefs about what the snake represented. What does this say about the power of their belief systems? Each of us has beliefs that have been shaped by our parents, teachers, the media, books, our culture, our experiences, and virtually everything that has happened in our lives. Our beliefs become the filter through which we view our world. Changing the health of our bodies almost always requires changing our beliefs about what affects us.

For example, a former patient with food allergies that became so obsessed by her reaction to food (believing that anything could provoke a reaction) that she eventually was unable to eat anything but rice and water. In this case, we had to work more closely with her beliefs around food. There are reports in the medical literature of allergic people who developed wheezing upon seeing an artificial flower.[19]

Psychologist and author Dr. Wayne Dyer talks extensively about becoming a "no limit person." What he means is that we constantly limit what we are able to accomplish by holding on to our "limiting" beliefs. Our goal should be to develop a belief system in which we do not limit ourselves.

For example, many people believe that with age comes infirmity, loss of mental faculties, weakness, tiredness, and loss of stamina. These are all limiting beliefs. Noted physician and author Deepak Chopra clearly makes this point in his book *Ageless Body, Timeless Mind*. If one believes that declining energy and function come with aging, this is how he or she will age.[20] The age really doesn't matter, either. I have seen patients who joke about their weight gain, muscle loss, sleepiness, fatigue, or whatever it may have been as "just due to old age." These were often people in their 30s, 40s, and 50s.

Scientists are completely rethinking what it means to age. People in their 80s and 90s have taken up mountain climbing, SCUBA diving, sky diving, hang gliding, and all manner of physically challenging sports. A 76-year-old man just ran across the United States, covering an average of 25 miles each day. A 92-year-old woman recently climbed Mount Fuji in Japan. An 85-year-old woman began SCUBA diving at 82 and recently dove the Great Barrier Reef in Australia. These people and others like them have shaken the limiting belief that with age comes declining energy and function.

Consider these three questions. Do not give them much thought. Write down the first thing that comes to mind.

Do you believe it is possible to get well?

Do you believe that *you* will ever be well?

Who is responsible for your health and wellness?

If the answer to the first two questions is "no," there is not much likelihood of healing until the belief is changed. This is because your biology follows your belief. Your physiology will take on the messages sent by your mind. If you answered with anyone other than yourself to the last question, you have a limiting belief that your health and wellness are in the hands of someone else, beyond your control. There is an old saying that goes "Believe you can or believe you cannot, either way you will be right." How true.

Remember, you are the healer. When you accept this belief you are better able to take charge of your healing. You no longer rely on an outside force. Certainly we all need people with expertise in the healing arts to help guide us on our healing journey. But this is what they are—guides.

Optimism

One of the most fascinating chapters in the mind-body story is the growing understanding of the role optimism plays in fostering good health. There is convincing evidence that optimists have more robust immune systems and that they suffer less illness in general than their pessimist counterparts. In his book *Who Gets Sick,* medical writer Blair Justice begins a section with the definition of a pessimist. He writes, "A pessimist is someone who, when confronted with two unpleasant alternatives, selects both."[21] Taking his definition a step further, you might say that an optimist is one who, when confronted with these alternatives chooses neither, diminishes their significance or finds the positive possibilities in each. *The American Heritage Dictionary* defines an optimist as one who usually expects a favorable outcome.

In an oft-cited study, researchers at the University of Michigan studied the effects of optimism/pessimism on the health of Harvard University graduates who were first interviewed in 1946 and followed for 35 years. Subjects were asked about difficult experiences encountered in World War II. The accounts were classified as global ("It will ruin my whole life"), stable ("It will never go away"), or internal ("It was all my fault"). Those with negative or pessimistic interpretations of their experiences were found to be consistently sicker than their more optimistic peers.[22]

The leader of this study, Dr. Christopher Peterson, listed a number of reasons why pessimism may contribute to more frequent illness:

- Pessimism may be linked to poor problem-solving ability and therefore to serious problems—hence, vulnerability to illness.
- Pessimism may lead to social withdrawal, behavior also associated with illness.
- Pessimism-related helplessness may affect immune function.

There is also direct evidence that optimists enjoy better immune function than pessimists. In their book *Healthy Pleasures*, David Sobel, M.D., and Robert Ornstein, Ph.D., report that when the blood of optimists is compared with that of pessimists, the optimists have higher levels of T-helper cells in relation to T-suppressors. Recall that T-helper cells stimulate immune function while T-suppressors suppress immune function. A high "helper" to "suppressor" ratio is desirable since resistance to infection and other illness would be enhanced.[23]

Martin Seligman, Ph.D., is Director of Clinical Training in Psychology at the University of Pennsylvania and is the leading researcher in the study of the effects of optimism on immune function. His observations after decades of extensive research include the following:[24]

- Pessimists make twice as many visits to the doctor as optimists.
- Pessimists have *twice* as many infectious diseases as optimists.
- Optimists have more active and more efficient immune systems.
- Pessimism often leads to depression, which causes a downturn in immune function.
- Major life changes can cause a decrease in immune function. In optimists the effects are less severe than in pessimists.
- Statistically, pessimists encounter more negative life events. The more bad life events we encounter, the more illness we will likely experience.

Seligman's observation that pessimists suffer more bad life events is stunning given the role bad life events play in illness. He states, "It has been shown statistically that the more bad events a person encounters in any given time period, the more illness he will have.... Who would you guess, encounters more bad events in life? Pessimists do. Because they are more passive, they are less likely to take steps to avoid bad events, and less likely to do anything to stop them once they start."[25]

Do pessimists suffer more frequently from chronic fatigue than optimists? Is it more common to be chronically tired if you are a pessimist? To date, the question has not been studied. However, optimism and pessimism have been studied in a variety of other illnesses and the consistent pattern appears to be that optimists suffer less illness in general regardless of the nature of the illness. Given the adverse effect of pessimism on immune function and the important role of the immune system in many patients who suffer from fatigue, it seems logical that we look at this critical psychological factor in any plan directed at improving health. In my clinical experience, patients who I might define as pessimists have seemed more resistant to successful treatment and less likely to experience full recovery than those I would categorize as optimists. This is true whether their primary complaint is recurrent respiratory infections, low back pain, allergies, headaches, chronic fatigue, or any number of others.

Questions always arise when talking about optimism and pessimism. "If I am a pessimist, is there any way to change?" Dr. Seligman's experience suggests that changing from a pessimist to an optimist (relatively speaking) can be accomplished by taking certain steps. These are described in his book *Learned Optimism*. Another question commonly offered is, "Is there an adverse health consequence to being overly optimistic?" Seligman also addresses this in his writings. There are certain risks associated with being *overly* optimistic. The key appears to be a healthy balance.

Seligman provides a questionnaire in his book to determine your explanatory style and learn whether you are an optimist or a pessimist. He then outlines a process by which you can begin to enhance your health by modifying your explanatory style. In my opinion, the reward available to the chronically tired person is well worth the cost and effort.

In Review

1. Psychological and behavioral factors can contribute to chronic fatigue and low vitality.
2. Depression is a common disorder with many different possible causes.
3. Some people with depression respond well to medication. Others are helped by modifying diet, nutrition, lifestyle, and environmental factors.
4. Stress can play a role in development of fatigue.
5. Stress, and the way in which you cope with stress, can adversely affect immune function, making one more susceptible to infection—another cause of fatigue.
6. Beliefs affect the way in which we look at events and can be a persistent contributor to low energy. Changing beliefs can often aid in improving energy.
7. The meaning our experiences hold for us and and possessing a sense of meaning and purpose are energizing forces.

8. Optimists tend to have more vibrant immune systems and suffer less illness in general than pessimists.

9. People who suffer from mood disorders should consider seeking professional help.

Chapter 23

Motherhood and Fatigue

MOTHERHOOD IS ONE of the most physically and emotionally demanding jobs a woman will ever perform. The stress of bodily changes, extra weight, nutritional demands, rapid weight loss, care giving, sleep deprivation, nursing, and changing family dynamics makes these periods especially challenging. Given these circumstances, it is no surprise that fatigue, tiredness, and exhaustion are among the most common symptoms that mothers report to their doctors.

If you are fatigued and your fatigue has set in during pregnancy or some time after the birth of your child, you will want to identify the factors that may be involved. Some possible causes of mother's fatigue are:

1. *Thyroid disorder.* Either overactive or underactive thyroid can cause fatigue. Decline in thyroid function may occur during the postpartum period and may persist for some time unless corrected. In one study, 7.2 percent of 293 women developed postpartum thyroid dysfunction.[1]

2. *Adrenal insufficiency.* As discussed earlier, the adrenal glands play an important role in maintaining energy. Adrenal exhaustion can occur in anyone due to a variety of factors, but the nutritional, physiological, and psychological stresses of pregnancy and motherhood often tax the adrenals to their limit. Adrenal insufficiency can

also contribute to postpartum depression. An assessment of adrenal cortisol and DHEA can reveal whether adrenal problems exist.

3. *Postpartum depression.* This is a common cause of fatigue among new mothers. It can be associated with poor thyroid function, sleep deprivation, isolation, nutrient deficiency, adrenal insufficiency, or other factors.

4. *Nutritional deficiency.* Deficiencies of certain nutrients may develop during pregnancy, during the postpartum period, and during lactation in breast feeding mothers. Some mothers become deficient in essential fatty acids, iron, zinc, or magnesium because of the demands of breast feeding. Each of these can contribute directly to fatigue. Magnesium and iron deficiency can further complicate matters because insomnia may develop.

Theoretically, any one of a number of nutrients can become deficient during pregnancy, during lactation, or during the child-raising years. Those listed below are somewhat common. For more information on signs, symptoms, and nutrient deficiencies associated with fatigue, see chapter 4.

Iron	Folic acid
Vitamin B_{12}	Magnesium
Vitamin B_6	Essential fatty acids
Zinc	Calcium
Thiamin	

Essential fatty acids deserve special attention because of the way in which the developing child essentially robs the mother of fatty acids to build the child's brain. Several studies have shown that the fatty acid status of pregnant mothers declines during pregnancy and further declines during the nursing period.

Dr. Monique Al and her colleagues studied long-chain fatty acids such as DHA in pregnant women. Her group found that the mother's blood levels of the fatty acid DHA declined during pregnancy and that they became worse with each successive pregnancy. Dr. Al's group concluded, "during pregnancy, maternal DHA is mobilized from a store that is not easily replenished after delivery. As a result, the maternal and neonatal [infant] DHA status diminishes with each subsequent pregnancy."

Dr. Ralph Holman, of the University of Minnesota, has also measured the blood fatty acids of women during normal pregnancies. Holman's group found that during pregnancy, the level ≠of omega-3 fatty acids fell considerably when compared with non pregnant women. The abnormal fatty acid profiles persisted for at least six weeks after delivery, at which time the study was terminated. It is possible that fatty acid inadequacy may have persisted much longer than six weeks postpartum.

In Dr. Holman's study, DHA was the most depressed being found at only thirty-five percent of its pre-pregnancy level. ALA, EPA, and DHA all further decreased during the postpartum period. His work suggests that during pregnancy the omega-3 fatty acid levels fall significantly and that low levels continue to persist after delivery.

This phenomenon may be linked, in part, to the high rates of depression in women compared with men. In fact, scientists at the National Institutes of Health now believe that depleted fatty acid reserves in mothers may be a critical link to understanding postpartum depression. Moreover, there are other disorders of adult women such as PMS that are associated with abnormal fatty acid levels. Chronic fatigue and chronic fatigue syndrome, which more often affect women, have also been found to be associated with abnormal fatty acid levels. Multiple sclerosis is more common among women and has been associated with fatty acid abnormalities.

The findings of Dr. Al and others may mean that women who have had children, even though they may not currently be pregnant, might need fatty acid supplementation to restore their depleted reserves. Adult women wishing to become pregnant should also ensure that their fatty acid status is at its peak.

While many of these studies focused on DHA, I believe that many doctors will agree that achieving a balance between GLA, ALA, DHA, and AA in adult women and during and after pregnancy is important. This can be achieved by supplemental doses of fish oil, DHA-rich oil, GLA-rich primrose oil, and ALA-rich flax seed oil. Since each pregnancy is unique and we are usually careful about supplementation during pregnancy, it may be wise to consult a health care professional to establish the right amounts for a given individual. This is especially true if the mother has a neurological disorder such as MS or seizures.

Mothers should also not adopt low-fat diets in order to lose weight after pregnancy. This can further worsen essential fatty acid deficiency. For more information on fatty acid nutrition and mental/emotional well being see *Smart Fats: How Dietary Fats and Oils Affect Mental, Physical, and Emotional Intelligence* (M.A. Schmidt, North Atlantic Books, 1997).

5. *Blood sugar disorders.* Hypoglycemia or diabetes may develop with the changing physiology brought about by bearing a child. Hypoglycemia is the more common of the two. The symptoms include:

Fatigue	Tiredness
Mood swings	Nervousness
Dizziness	Rapid heart beat (some)

Symptoms typically begin three to five hours after a meal. If they begin within zero to three hours of a meal, consider food allergy or a high tryptophan/high carbohydrate diet as the cause.

6. *Diet.* Because of fatigue and time constraints, some mothers do not consume foods that are optimum with regard to nutrient content. Overconsumption of convenience foods can also lead to problems. Make consumption of nutrient-rich foods a priority and avoid processed and packaged foods as much as possible. Note that nursing mothers who are vegetarians have a high likelihood of developing vitamin B_{12} deficiency.

7. *Family stress.* Motherhood can also contribute to fatigue because of the enormous changes in relationships and family dynamics that occur with the introduction of a new life into the family.

Signs and Symptoms

The signs and symptoms of fatigue associated with parenting may cover the entire spectrum of topics discussed in this book. If you have specific symptoms that fit any of the conditions mentioned in previous chapters, you should have an examination to confirm the presence or absence of such a condition.

Laboratory Tests

Fatigue of motherhood may be associated with any one of a number of medical problems. General screening tests are usually used initially. More sophisticated tests follow if the cause cannot be detected with basic tests. Common preliminary tests include:

- SMAC
- CBC with differential
- Serum ferritin (for iron status)
- Thyroid panel
- Tests for B_{12} and folic acid status.
- Tests for other vitamins and minerals
- Salivary cortisol and DHEA
- Essential fatty acids (red blood cell)

Treatment

The first step in dealing with fatigue of motherhood is to visit your doctor and rule out any medical conditions that may be causing your fatigue. These might include thyroid disorders, depression, low blood sugar, diabetes, adrenal insufficiency, or more serious conditions.

An evaluation of your nutritional status should be a high priority because many nutrients may be influenced by pregnancy, lactation, and the stress of parenthood. Nutrient supplementation is extremely helpful in fatigue of motherhood.

Many mothers do not get adequate exercise because they often cannot find the time. Exercise of some form should be a priority. It improves endurance and stamina, improves energy metabolism, can remedy depression, and serves as a social outlet.

Get extra sleep. This of course is a luxury of which every mother dreams, more easily said than done. Nevertheless, every effort should be made to improve the quantity and quality of sleep. Relaxation exercises, deep breathing, yoga, visualization, and self-hypnosis are all techniques that can be used to improve sleep quality.

In Review

1. Fatigue is a common occurrence among mothers.

2. Possible causes include thyroid problems, inadequate diet, nutritional deficiency, relationship changes, blood sugar problems, depression, and sleep apnea.

3. Various medical conditions may also produce fatigue.

4. Exercise, adequate rest, good nutrition, and family support are key ingredients to improving energy.

Part II

Steps to Improved Energy

Chapter 24

Boosting Energy and Restoring Balance

DOCTORS AND PATIENTS often become obsessed with finding a single cause for an ailment. There is a prevailing belief in medicine that if a certain set of symptoms exists, then a specific drug, nutrient, remedy, surgery, or treatment must be given. Specific treatments remain a vital part of health care. However, it is important to consider that much illness arises out of imbalance rather than because of a specific thing. By restoring balance, many of the maladies that afflict modern humans can be remedied. This idea is based on research and borne out by clinical experience.

I have seen a significant number of patients report near-miraculous recoveries by changing how they live, eat, behave, and view life—in essence, by restoring balance. Tracy was a 35-year-old mother of two with severe debilitating fatigue and headaches. During her initial exam in my office she told me that she had said these words in a prayer the previous night: "Dear God, please end my life and give my husband a wife who can better care for my two girls." She had seen many doctors over the years with little success. Her medical file was eight inches thick. Tracy was desperate and felt as though she had exhausted her options. We did many things in the course of her treatment, most of which were focused on restoring balance. I'm convinced that what made the greatest difference was the dietary, attitude, and lifestyle changes made by Tracy.

Evidence of the need for balance pervades the medical literature. If we don't consume enough calories, our immune systems falter and we succumb to infection. Yet, if we consume calories in excess, our immune systems falter as well. This was shown at the Massachusetts Institute of Technology when overfed dogs were more likely to become infected and develop encephalitis from canine distemper virus infection.[1]

Exercise provides another example. Those who don't exercise are, in general, more apt to get a variety of illnesses. Included are sluggish immunity and increased infection susceptibility.[2] On the other hand, those who exercise excessively or who overtrain can suppress their immunity and easily succumb to infection. In fact, elite athletes and runners are more susceptible to infections than the average person.[3]

In general, people who are married live longer and have fewer health problems than those who are single.[4] However, when one forms an intimate relationship there is always a risk of losing that person. The death of a spouse can lead to a significant decline in immune function and be followed by illness or death in the surviving spouse.

The need for balance is even reflected in the world of work. People who have no job often feel depressed and suffer from lack of meaning and purpose. This can be enormously stressful and may lead to poor health or disease. Yet people with jobs who are overworked may become "burned out," depressed, and may even die of a heart attack.

Some may interpret this as, "Well, everything is bad for you. Eat too much—get sick, eat too little—get sick. Exercise too much—get sick, exercise too little—get sick. Work too much—get sick, no work—get sick." But this is not the message at all. The message is that moderation and balance may be important aspects of maintaining health. When we lead a life of extremes, imbalance may more easily occur. The key, I believe, is to combine a life of balanced being with a life of passion, zest, and meaningful pursuit.

Throughout this book, I've discussed a number of specific contributors to fatigue, tiredness, and low vitality. Addressing one or more of these factors may be important and necessary to ultimately attaining the level of health you desire. However, it may also be possible for you to overcome your fatigue (or at least improve your energy) not by specific means, but by a general effort to restore balance to all aspects of your life. Before you embark on a complicated trek to seek out the cause of your fatigue, you may want to try a series of basic strategies designed to help boost energy.

1. *Exercise = Energy.* Have you ever wondered how those people who exercise seem to have so much energy? It is not because they naturally have more energy, it is because exercise gives them more energy. Anyone who has exercised knows that they feel more energized at the end of a workout than at the beginning. It seems almost paradoxical, but when you drag yourself home from a hard day and plop into the couch, what you really need is a session of walking, aerobics, golf, running, or whatever physical activity you enjoy.

You need not engage in intensely strenuous physical activity to derive benefit. Moderate exercise such as walking for one hour, four to five times each week, confers many health dividends. Remember, there is a difference between exercising to maintain health and exercising to become physically fit.

If you have been diagnosed with chronic fatigue syndrome, or if you suffer from cardiovascular disease or another health condition, you must approach exercise with caution. See your doctor about the best way to begin.

2. *Eat food that optimizes your mood.* If you need to be alert for an afternoon meeting, do not eat fettucini Alfredo with a rich cheese and butter sauce. The starch may lead to more serotonin production, which triggers sleepiness and relaxation. The fat will slow digestion and divert more blood to the gut, away from the brain. Remember the chapter on food and mood. If you want to be alert, consume foods that are low in fat and contain some protein. Fruits and vegetables are essentially mood-neutral, so have as many of these as you like (except for starchy foods like potatoes).

3. *Stretch every day.* Stretching and flexibility exercises help to move blood and lymph throughout the body and prevent stagnation. They improve your oxygen transport to the brain and other

tissues and can have an enormous positive effect on your energy. If you incorporate stretching movements that involve the spinal column, you increase the benefit greatly since flexion and extension of the spine stimulate one of the largest networks of veins in the body.

Yoga is an excellent exercise to stimulate energy. It incorporates body movement with stretching of muscles and deep breathing. Deep breathing is another way to increase your energy and feeling of wellbeing.

4. *Deep breathing.* Deep breathing exercises are an excellent means to boost energy. Deep breathing exercises also lower the level of stress hormones circulating in your body. Most of us breathe shallowly and from the chest. Breathing should originate in the abdomen. As you breathe, you should observe the rise and fall of your tummy with each breath.

Organisms that live the longest on this planet have the slowest rates of breathing. It seems that most mammals take roughly the same number of breaths in their lifetime. Those with higher metabolic rates that breathe more often live shorter lives. Those that breathe more slowly live longer. The average adult breathes about 12 to 20 times each minute. Those who take full advantage of slow, rhythmic, deep breathing breathe only about four to eight times each minute and still provide the body with optimum oxygen.

Take five to ten minutes each day to do deep breathing exercises. Also, take note of your breathing throughout the day. Notice whether you are taking shallow breaths and in what circumstances. Many people become tense and take shallow breaths while under stress or thinking about something urgent or stressful. These are precisely the times when deep breathing is most needed.

5. *Meditation.* Deep breathing exercises are the first step to truly finding a balance point within yourself. The next step is meditation. Meditation has a different meaning for different people. For our purpose it can mean emptying the mind of thoughts, images, expectations, chatter, noise, and the day-to-day ramblings on which our mind embarks. In doing so, we are better able to listen to signs and cues our body is sending about our deeper needs. Many patients find that joining a meditation group is helpful because they are

guided through the steps and helped by the supportive atmosphere.

For those of you who think that meditation is still a fringe activity, be aware that many hospitals now offer meditation classes to their patients as a means to reduce surgical complications, speed recovery, improve healing, reduce anxiety, and improve the overall quality of medical care.

5. *Get it off your chest.* Emotional distress can sap your energy as quickly as almost anything. If you hold the emotions within, failing to express them to anyone, the drain on your energy becomes even greater. Whether you wrestle with marital problems, a toxic mate, an obnoxious boss, unruly kids, or the like, how you cope with it dictates the impact it will have on your mood and energy. You can think of this as emotional baggage that you carry around with you. Imagine that your car is loaded with suitcases, and the rear end sags close to the ground. Now imagine that your car is approaching a uphill climb. You are already loaded to the maximum. Now you trudge up the hill slowly, laboriously, and burning gallons of fuel. Our emotional baggage can act much like this. By unloading our baggage, by sharing our feelings with someone we trust (or journaling if there is no one you trust), we lighten the load, use less fuel, and make the journey easier.

6. *Find your rhythm.* Each of us has biological rhythms that are similar. Then again, we are all individuals with individual idiosyncrasies. For example, you may be a "night person" while your sibling or neighbor is a "morning person." The night person is wide awake at 11:00 P.M. and performs his best work at that time. Yet when 6:00 A.M. rolls around, he's nowhere to be found, barely functioning. The morning person, much to the chagrin of many of us, rises blissfully at 5:30 A.M., throws on the jogging shorts, and darts out the door whistling. He is bright and alert at the 8:00 A.M. office briefing while most others are slurping their third cup of coffee to stay awake. However, the morning person often fizzles out by 10:00 P.M., ready for bed.

Look carefully at your own rhythms. Note when you are always up, and when you're down. What are your peak performing hours and when are you normally less productive? Once you have determined this, plan your activities accordingly. I do some of my best writing after 10:00 P.M. Sometimes I can sit and stare at the computer for hours in the morning with little inspiration. Yet at night, the ideas often flow freely.

Also look at your work situation. If you sit at a desk all day long and feel fatigue or tiredness setting in, you may want to get up and walk around the office or go for a walk outside.

7. Some of the greatest achievers in history were notorious nappers—Benjamin Franklin and Leonardo Da Vinci, to mention just two. A *ten- or fifteen-minute* nap at lunchtime or in mid-afternoon may be a welcome boost to both body and intellect. Just don't make the nap so long that it interferes with restful sleep at night. This mid-afternoon sojourn may be a good time to find a quiet place and do some deep breathing exercises.

8. *Evaluate your sleep needs.* If you're tired, it may mean that you do not get enough sleep at night. Try going to bed at 10:00 instead of 10:30 or 11:00 and see if the extra sleep helps. Follow the rules for better sleep mentioned elsewhere in this book. If you suffer from insomnia, look carefully at the chapter on sleep. If you still can't solve the problem, see a sleep disorders specialist.

9. *Avoid the "three squares."* The habit of eating three square meals a day is an American tradition. However, many doctors are beginning to believe that eating five or six small meals a day is much better than eating three large meals a day. It helps maintain your blood sugar and energy at a more even level. Also, digestion requires a lot of your blood supply, especially if the meal is heavy. That means less blood for the brain, which can lead to tiredness and sluggish mental ability. Studies have also shown that rats raised on six meals a day live longer than those raised on three a day, even if the total calories are the same.

10. *Attitude.* Our attitudes greatly influence how we feel. Optimists have been shown to have more active immune systems, experience less illness, make fewer trips to the doctor, and experience fewer negative life events. If you see yourself as somewhat of a pessimist, you may wish to work on changing your outlook.

11. *Sugar and processed foods.* Eliminate refined sugar for at least

two months. Avoid adding sugar to your coffee, cereal, and other foods. Avoid sugared cereals, candies, pastries, and other snack foods. Read labels and avoid foods that list any sugar as one of the top six ingredients. Agree to do this for two months. If after two months it seems to have made no difference, you may go back to your old ways (though reducing sugar has many other benefits). Remember, the average American consumes roughly 120 pounds of sugar each year. Many people find that reducing the amount of sugar consumed gives them a tremendous boost of energy.

12. *Caffeine, aspartame, and alcohol.* These are known to cause fatigue in some people. Reduce your intake of these three (if you now consume them) for three to four weeks. Eliminating them entirely would be ideal. See if it makes a difference. You might be surprised at the surge in energy you experience.

13. *Massage.* Therapeutic massage can be a valuable part of any effort to boost energy and restore balance. Massage can improve immunity, promote circulation, improve digestion, reduce muscle tension, reduce the stress response, stimulate the elimination of metabolic toxins that build up in body tissues, and stimulate the nervous system. It also satisfies a need for touch that is inherent in every human being.

14. *Laugh.* It is amazing how energizing laughter can be. Laughter reduces stress hormone levels, increases immune function, improves circulation, and activates certain muscle groups as though they had been through an exercise session. Instead of watching the nightly news and all the violence-oriented programs, vow only to watch programs that are funny or enlightening. Perhaps you might even discontinue reading the newspaper for one month to get a break from the daily tidings of bad news.

15. *Reach out to others.* Those who live in isolation suffer more depression, illness, and early death than those with close social ties. One can live among others and be emotionally isolated. One can also live in an isolated area with insufficient contact with friends, neighbors, or relatives. Neither situation is optimum for good health. Find individuals with whom you can interact and share. It may mean attending events, joining groups, or asking for friendship. Humans

are by nature social creatures. We are entirely interdependent upon one another. Our lives are often what we make of them.

16. *Build your muscles.* To many of us in the field of functional medicine it is obvious, but to most people the importance of muscle is not well understood. Your muscles are the engines that burn calories in your body to generate energy. When your lean muscle mass is too low, you lack the machinery to burn the calories you must. Thus, you produce less energy.

You should make every effort to reduce your percentage of body fat (if it is excessive) and increase your lean muscle mass. Go to a clinic that will measure your percent body fat. It should be between 15 and 22 percent, depending upon your age and sex. You then want to set out on a program that will lower body fat and build muscle. Building muscle means combining aerobic exercise with weight-bearing exercises that push the muscle beyond its normal limit. Don't be afraid if you've never done this. Studies with 80-year-old people have shown that even at this age muscle mass can be increased significantly in only six weeks.

17. *Fun and play.* One of the critical elements left out of many health-related books is the importance of fun and play. In my opinion, without fun and play this whole business of life takes on far too somber a tone. Many people complain that they do not have "time" to play. In our busy, overly serious world, we must plan our play. Take a period of each day and set it aside for some kind of play. This would preferably be outdoors since we also lack outdoor exposure to fresh air and light. Playing outdoors would accomplish all of these. If you have children, try to get down to their level. There are no greater teachers of play than children.

18. *Quality and quantity of water.* Many water supplies are now contaminated with toxins. Even chlorine and fluoride that are added to city water supplies can contribute to or aggravate health problems. Make sure you drink pure water. Then you must drink the water, at least eight glasses each day. Juice, coffee, pop, and tea do not count. You must drink water. If you don't drink enough you don't detoxify as well.

The work of Dr. F. Batmanghelhidj in an Iranian prisoner of war camp, illustrates the dramatic effect water consumption can have on health. He was surrounded by prisoners who were sick from a wide range of diseases. A prisoner himself, he had no medicine to treat these men—only water. By administering water, he was able to restore health in seemingly incurable conditions. This was astonishing to a physician accustomed to using drugs as treatment. He has continued his research and has worked out numerous biochemical mechanisms for the effect of water on health. In essence, increasing water intake normalizes physiology and biochemistry in measurable ways. His book *Your Body's Many Cries for Water,* is a fascinating account about how water improves health.[5]

19. *Fresh air.* Get outdoors and breathe fresh air as often as you can. Fresh air can be enormously invigorating. When you are in the fresh air, remember to breathe deeply. If you live in the city, get out to the country often. Polluted air is filled with chemical oxidants that slowly deplete our antioxidant stores. Avoid exercising in polluted environments.

20. *Recognize the seasons.* In nature there are seasons—winter, spring, summer, fall. In life there are seasons—infancy, childhood, adolescence, adulthood, middle age, the elder years. The seasons involve natural changes to which each of us must adapt. Likewise, I believe, there are seasons of health. As we move through life, our bodies change and adapt to the circumstances that surround us. In response, we too must adapt. We must recognize that these seasons of health may also carry messages for us. If you suffer from a health problem, see if perhaps you are amidst a change in season, and ask yourself what you might do to optimize your passage through that season.

Because each of us is unique, the activities that collectively provide us with a balanced life will vary. For any given person the activities may vary based on the season, the time of life, cycles of business, relationships, and many other factors. A worthy goal is to develop the skill of listening to your body's signals to learn what it needs at any particular time. You might find that during winter you need to go to bed earlier; during the flu you need to eat less; when you have a headache you need to read less, think less, and watch less television; when you have a sore throat you may have unspoken words that need to be expressed; when you have a busy schedule that confines you to the office or the desk you may need extra exercise; when you've been traveling out of town you may need to spend extra time with your family to restore balance.

Rigid routines and self-imposed inflexible rules are not the means to optimal health. Healthy choices arise out of having a set of sensible, flexible, healthy guidelines coupled with an inner voice that helps us navigate through the inevitable sea of change that is life.

Chapter 25

Detoxification

THROUGHOUT THIS BOOK I have discussed the fatigue-inducing effects of such things as chemical toxicity, prescription drugs, intestinal dysbiosis, chronic stress, insufficient hydration (water), food allergy, food additives, environmental allergens, hidden infections, overweight/underlean, and other factors. Added to this is nutritional insufficiency, which aggravates each of the above conditions (and in many cases precedes or is a result of them).

A common theme that underlies each of the above concerns it that of toxicity. Prescription drugs may add to the toxic burden. Chemicals in the environment add to the toxic burden. The products of intestinal putrefaction and fermentation add to the burden. Stress hormones circulating in the bloodstream add to the burden, as do the other factors mentioned. These factors can act alone to cause fatigue or they may act in concert. More often than not, they act in concert to create what is called the total toxic load.

The total toxic load is often sufficient to disrupt the normal activities of cellular metabolism, which then alters energy production. Nutrient insufficiency contributes to poor energy production as well. Moreover, nutrient insufficiency renders the body's normal detoxication pathways less efficient. The combination of body toxicity and nutrient insufficiency leads to a situation in which the cells and tissues are burdened by toxins, but unable to readily remove them because of impaired elimination mechanisms brought on by insufficient nutrient levels.

The cost of this dynamic interaction may be poor energy production and disrupted function of the immune system, endocrine system, nervous system, inflammatory system, circulatory system, and potentially any other body system (depending on the person's biochemical uniqueness). Some researchers working with fatigued patients have moved away from the search for a single cause and recognize that an accumulation of factors is more likely responsible for the condition. Their approach has been to direct efforts at detoxification and improving nutrient utilization. The theory is that by encouraging elimination of toxins from the tissues, the body will begin to function more efficiently on its own. Once functioning efficiently, energy production improves and fatigue is eliminated.

One who has pioneered this concept is Jeffrey Bland, Ph.D., of Gig Harbor, Washington. In 1991, Bland introduced a medical food developed for the purposes of detoxification. The formula is a rice-based, low-allergen mixture with a wide range of macro- and micronutrients designed to enhance liver function and promote detoxification of accumulated toxins from the body.

Bland and Rigden reported on their study of 36 people with chronic fatigue who underwent therapy using their program. Before beginning the program, each person was asked to complete a symptom survey, which was scored according to the number and severity of symptoms. The average initial score was 173. After only one month, there was a 50 percent reduction in symptoms. After three months on the program the average score had fallen to 77. A maintenance program was continued and most patients experienced continued improvement in not only fatigue symptoms, but other symptoms as well.[1]

According to *Casarett and Doull's Toxicology,* fatigue is associated with chronic toxicity.[2] Other symptoms of chronic toxicity include alterations of the immune and neurological systems. According to Bland, chronic exposure to toxins could result in metabolic "poisoning" and impairment of the body's energy pathways, producing fatigue, muscle weakness, lassitude, and immune and endocrine symptoms.[3]

One common finding among fatigued people is low levels of magnesium in the cells. In many such cases, oral supplementation with magnesium is not adequate to raise the cellular levels of magnesium. This is because moving magnesium from outside the cell to inside the cell requires energy (ATP). Yet many fatigued patients suffer from poor ATP, or energy production. It is a "catch-22." Magnesium is needed to produce ATP, but ATP is needed to get magnesium into the cell where it can be used. Toxicity is thought to be one reason the energy production is disrupted. In Rigden and Bland's study, when the detoxification program was implemented, cellular magnesium levels improved. They concluded, "The results of this study suggest strongly that many of the symptoms of metabolic disturbances observed in the chronic fatigue patient can be improved by a nutritional intervention program utilizing enhanced levels of specific nutrients recognized to support improved hepatic [liver] detoxification."[4]

Signs and Symptoms

The signs and symptoms that might indicate toxicity include any of those mentioned in this book. The most common complaints are chronic fatigue and low vitality.

Laboratory Tests

Tests to assess toxicity have been discussed in previous chapters. The primary ones we're concerned with here are functional liver tests and tests for toxic exposure.

- *Caffeine clearance (saliva)*. Assesses the activity of an aspect of a liver detoxication enzyme system known as cytochrome P450.
- *Benzoate loading (urine)*. Assesses the activity of the second phase of liver detoxication.
- *D-glucaric acid (urine)*. Reflects exposure to toxic compounds.
- *Mercapturic acid (urine)*. Reflects exposure to toxic compounds.
- *Blood levels* of toxic organic substances.

Treatment

Detoxification involves several key steps.

1. Identification and elimination of reactive foods, chemicals, additives, and other substances.

2. Consumption of a diet low in reactive or allergic foods.

3. Detoxification program for seven to twenty-one days.

4. Low-temperature sauna. This is being used by some doctors to encourage elimination of fat-soluble toxins through the skin.

5. Nutrition support that includes antioxidants and detoxification cofactors.

6. Support the endocrine, immune, and hepatic (liver) system.

7. Begin a program of behavioral therapy and stress management.

8. Restore gastrointestinal function.

Because of the growing awareness of the role of toxicity in illness, more doctors and health advocates are beginning to offer various detoxification programs. It will be difficult for the consumer to know how many of these are safe and effective. I am personally concerned about people who advocate strict fasting as a form of detoxification. Fasting has many benefits. However, for the purposes of detoxifying, the lack of nutrients may be problematic. As the body begins to detoxify, it releases toxins that have been stored in fat cells for many years. As these toxins are released they must be processed by the liver and kidneys. This requires a host of antioxidant nutrients and a very active liver detoxication system (which is heavily nutrient-dependent). Purging your fat stores of toxins can result in reexposure and toxic damage if your nutrient status is not optimum. Average levels will not suffice in a detoxification program. The levels must be higher than normal.

Another important consideration is that glutathione, one of the body's most critical compounds for detoxication, is formed from three amino acids (cysteine, glycine, and glutamic acid). These amino acids can be obtained from the diet. Cysteine is more typically the one that is deficient and is called the rate-limiting amino acid of glutathione formation. During fasting states, inadequate levels of these amino acids are consumed and insufficient glutathione is made. Thus, poor detoxication may occur.

Various types of detoxification programs are being used successfully. Dr. Bland's UltraClear Metabolic Clearing Therapy is only one. Sherry Rogers, M.D., who is a pioneer in the treatment of chemically sensitive and chronically ill patients, successfully uses a modification of the macrobiotic diet. William Rea, M.D., a leader in the field of environmental medicine and director of the Environmental Health Center in Dallas, Texas, relies on a complex formula of environmental control, nutrient supplementation, sauna depurition, desensitization, endocrine therapy, avoidance, and behavior therapy. Russell Jaffe, M.D., Ph.D., of the Health Studies Collegium, identifies immunotoxins, using a lymphocyte response assay, and removes them from the patient's environment. Nutritional protocols aimed at immune repair are then used to enhance defenses.

The current therapies are, I believe, only a hint of what will come in this rapidly expanding and complex field of metabolic detoxification. It is truly an exciting time because it represents a merging of many fascinating disciplines and offers hope and healing to a broad range of people who may have had previously intractable disorders.

Chapter 26

Breath and Energy

THE BREATH IS ONE of the most powerful energizing forces we have. When we breathe deeply, we bring oxygen-rich air deep into our lungs to be distributed throughout the body. Oxygen is critical to the generation of energy within our cells. It is critical to our feeling of wellbeing. We can live without food for weeks, without water for days, but without air for only minutes.

I have observed that many people who suffer from fatigue and low vitality are shallow breathers. They take only partial breaths, breathe too often, and breathe with their chest rather than their abdomen. In order to get an optimum amount of oxygen into the tissues you must breathe slowly, rhythmically, and deeply. Most people take twelve to twenty breaths each minute. In order to do this, breathing must be shallow and rapid. The lungs are never allowed to fill completely with air. It is possible to breathe only four to eight times each minute. When you breathe at this rate your stress levels begin to fall, stress hormones decrease, sleep improves, cell energy metabolism improves, and emotional health improves. Organ health also improves.

In addition, the depth of your breathing is directly related to your emotional state and your energy. When you breathe more deeply and slowly, the release of pent-up feelings begins to occur. Shallow breathing almost always accompanies distressed emotional states.

By developing proper breathing techniques, almost anyone can improve energy and vitality. There are many techniques available that help to optimize your breathing and improve energy. At the most basic level you might do two things. First, set aside ten minutes each day (fifteen to thirty minutes would be ideal) where you sit quietly with no distractions. Breathe in slowly to a count of eight. Your belly should move outward as you breathe in. Your chest, jaw, and shoulders should barely move. This ensures diaphragmatic breathing. Then let your breath out slowly to a count of eight as your belly moves inward, as though it were being drawn into your spine.

Your mind should focus only on the sound of the air rushing in and out of your mouth. Empty your mind of all thoughts and distractions. This may seem difficult at first, but if you remember to always draw your focus back to the sound of your breath it will be easier. Repeat the breathing cycles for ten to thirty minutes.

The second part of this simple approach involves awareness. Throughout the day, be aware of how you are breathing. If you find yourself breathing shallowly or sucking in your gut to look trim, shift immediately to slow, rhythmic diaphragmatic breaths where your belly rises and falls with each breath. As you improve your awareness and grow accustomed to breathing this way, it will become more automatic.

A more detailed approach, and one that has a more profound impact on body and emotions is a practice called Chi Kung. Chi Kung is a centuries-old practice developed in the Orient. It is used in many Chinese hospitals to improve energy and wellbeing and has become an important tool of many Western doctors and healers who practice mind/body medicine. Mantak Chia is one of several noted teachers of Chi Kung in the United States. He has written of a technique known as the "six healing sounds."[2,3] The six healing sounds are designed to balance and restore energy in the body. It is much like an internal massage that creates an energy flow in once-stagnant organs and tissues. In the process, it allows for the release of pent-up emotions and feelings that are so often a source of illness and fatigue.

William Collinge, Ph.D., who has created a mind/body program for people with CFS, recommends the six healing sounds exercises to his clients with chronic fatigue.³ He reports that it is simple to do and the results are significant. My own experience has been similar.

The six healing sounds exercise is best done in one session. Sit in a comfortable chair with your spine straight on the edge of your seat and your feet flat on the floor. Each sound is repeated six, nine, twelve, or twenty-four times. The sound is made on the exhaled breath. The exhaled breath should be long and slow, and you should empty your lungs as thoroughly as you can. Begin with the lung sound. In between each sound, rest, breathe, and quietly reflect.

1. *The lung sound.* Place your tongue behind your teeth and with a long slow exhalation make the "SSSSS" sound, as in "hiss." As you do this, imagine that your lungs are releasing grief, sadness, or depression. Picture these energies being released through your breath, as if they are a cloud being exhaled from the lungs. Imagine that your lungs are being filled with feelings of courage and righteousness.

After a series of breaths, rest silently for a few moments, then move on to the kidney sound.

2. *The kidney sound.* Form your lips in an "O" shape. As you slowly exhale make the sound "WOOOOO" as if you were blowing out a candle. The sound is made with the breath, not with the voice. As you make this sound, imagine that you are exhaling fear that has gathered in your kidneys. Picture the fear coming out like a cloud, being released from your kidneys. Imagine the fear is replaced by a feeling of gentleness.

Rest for a time, still imagining the kidneys making this sound. Then move to the liver sound.

3. *The liver sound.* Make a long, slow exhalation with the sound "SHHHHH" and imagine that anger is being released from the liver in the form of a cloud. The breath draws anger from the liver and exhales it in the form of a cloud. As the anger is emptied, fill the liver with feelings of kindness.

Rest silently, while imagining the liver is continuing to make this sound.

4. *The heart sound.* Open your mouth wide. With a long, slow exhalation make the sound "HAWWWWW" as in "*hawk*." Once again, the sound is made not with the voice, but with the rush of air. Imagine any feeling of impatience, hate, or arrogance being exhaled from the heart. Imagine the heart being filled with feelings of love, joy, and happiness.

Rest silently, while imagining that the heart is continuing to make this sound.

5. *The spleen sound.* Place your tongue against your palate and with a long slow exhalation make the "WHOOOO" sound. This sound is more guttural and throaty than the kidney sound. It should originate in your chest. The sound is made with the rush of air, not your voice. As you exhale, imagine a cloud of worry and anxiety is drifting from your spleen and out through your mouth. Imagine the spleen being filled with feelings of fairness.

Rest silently.

6. *The "triple warmer" sound.* This sound is done while lying quietly on your back. With the rush of air through your mouth, make a "HEEEEE" sound. As you slowly exhale, imagine a large rolling pin flattening out your body from head to toe. The rolling pin is rebalancing all the energies activated by the other sounds, and helps harmonize the energies of the three large areas of the body.

Rest quietly for ten minutes and imagine all the muscles and organs in your body in a relaxed state.

The healing sounds can have a profound balancing effect on the body and a calming effect on the nervous system. This can be done daily. A good time is just before bed.

Please don't underestimate the power of the breath to vitalize and energize your body and mind. I can almost guarantee that you will experience improved wellbeing and energy by combining two basic practices of the energizing breath:

1. A daily period of ten to thirty minutes of deep breathing, mind-calming, relaxation exercises.

2. Shifting your average rate of respiration during the day to six to ten breaths per minute with slow, abdominal breathing.

You can use the techniques described in this book or consult one of many other excellent books on the subject and find a method that suits your needs.

Chapter 27

Doing Your Detective Work:
Tests that Help Unravel the Mystery

MANY PEOPLE WHO suffer from chronic fatigue and low vitality travel from doctor to doctor in hopes that someone will solve the riddle of their poor health. In some cases, these pursuits are fruitful. In others, they may not be. Hopefully, this book has given you new insights into the possible contributors to your fatigue—factors that may have been previously overlooked.

Even though we have many new insights, there are substantial numbers of patients with chronic fatigue whose illnesses are very difficult to understand. The treatments are not as effective as doctors would like. There is more being learned each week about treating these difficult cases. The truth is, however, we have much, much more to learn. For those of you with a resistant case of chronic fatigue, I would like to take this chapter to discuss just one difficult case and then review a number of tests that may help in unraveling the mystery of your fatigue.

The Case of Dr. Tom

Tom was a doctor with a busy suburban practice in the Minneapolis area. He developed chronic fatigue in 1993, which led to slow and painful changes in his business and personal lives. He had gone from seeing patients five days a week to only three mornings a week. His physical activity was sharply restricted and he began to experience notable psychological changes. Tom sought the help of numerous health care professionals including a neurologist, internist, endocrinologist, infectious disease specialist, chiropractic nutritionist, and acupuncturist. Each of these was a reasonable choice and each professional undoubtedly had success treating patients with fatigue. Unfortunately, none was able to provide relief or obtain a reasonable understanding of what was wrong. Finally, the infectious disease expert determined that Tom had Lyme disease, an infection by the bacteria *Borrelia burdorferi*. Dr. Tom also showed evidence of infection by Epstein-Barr virus. He was placed on an extensive course of antibiotic in an effort to eradicate the bacterial infection. While antibiotics seemed to provide temporary relief from some symptoms, Tom's case proved to be generally resistant to treatment. He felt as though he were at a dead end with no insight as to what was wrong or where to go next.

I suggested that Tom take an entirely different view of his problem. I said, "We know that the bacterial and viral infections have taken place, but let's focus our efforts on your disrupted metabolism." It was my belief that he had to restore integrity to his immune defenses. I felt that if we looked closely at vitamin and mineral metabolism, amino acids, organic acids, essential fatty acids, toxic minerals, intestinal permeability, immune function, and other factors that we would be able to see where his body was not functioning and why. With this information, we might devise a treatment strategy that restored normal function—a strategy geared for long-term success—rather than one that focused on merely improving his symptoms in the short term.

The laboratory assessment I suggested included numerous tests for metabolic function and nutrient status. A comprehensive digestive stool analysis (CDSA) revealed significant intestinal dysbiosis (overgrowth of microbes in the gut). The analysis of red blood cells for trace minerals showed deficiency of magnesium and chromium, both involved in energy metabolism. Toxic metal analysis of hair revealed aluminum excess. His immune system showed low numbers of natural killer cells. Liver function tests showed he was not detoxifying properly. An organic acid analysis of his urine showed that he was deficient in B-vitamins including thiamin, riboflavin, niacin, pantothenic acid, and again, magnesium. He had elevated secretory IgA, which suggested an inflammatory or infectious process.

The amino acid taurine was low in his blood and high in his urine, indicating he was spilling this amino acid. Two amino acids (anserine and carnosine) showed up in his urine that indicated digestive enzyme inadequacy traceable to zinc deficiency. Amino acid analysis also showed evidence of vitamin B_{12} deficiency, a common occurrence among fatigued patients. Further analysis of his amino acids showed deficiency of tryptophan and cysteine, involved in neurotransmitter formation and detoxication respectively. He was also low in essential amino acids lysine, valine, tyrosine, arginine, histidine, and aspartic acid. Several amino acid abnormalities suggested B_6 and magnesium deficiency. Others suggested intestinal malabsorption.

What is most interesting about Dr. Tom's results is that his standard lab tests were essentially *normal*. He lived the experience of many patients. He felt lousy most of the time and knew there was something seriously wrong. Yet the tests said he was fine, other than an infection. After this evaluation, Tom felt that he finally had an explanation for what was wrong with him. More importantly, the information could be used to devise a treatment plan that was specifically tailored to his individual biochemical needs. Not only did Tom now have hope, but he had a powerful therapeutic tool to use in his recovery.

His therapeutic program consisted of the following:

> Intravenous vitamin C—25 grams twice a week.
> Oral vitamin C—26 to 10 grams daily to bowel tolerance.

Vitamin B_{12}	Magnesium
Chromium	Vitamin B_6
EPA (from fish oil)	Acidophilus and bifidus
Germanium	supplements
UltraClear Sustain	

Amino acids including:

Arginine	Glutamine
Histidine	Isoleucine
Leucine	Lysine
Phenylalanine	Taurine
Threonine	Tryptophan
Tyrosine	Valine

Exercise

Extra sleep

He continued to take the antibiotic once a day while on this program. His comment to me was, "It seems that the antibiotic doesn't help unless I am on the nutritional protocols. The vitamin C and essential fatty acids have been especially helpful." Dr. Tom felt that "the antibiotic helped bring the infection down to the point where the immune system could rebuild itself." Dr. Tom also felt that increasing the amount of daily sleep and increasing his exercise level have been invaluable components of his recovery.

It has been an uphill struggle for Tom. He spent nearly one year (prior to our encounter) on a drug-oriented treatment approach with only modest improvement. The specially tailored nutrition protocol based on his new lab reports has given him consistent improvement. The key to keep in mind is that this program was tailored to his biochemistry. He now feels that his treatment efforts are directed at correction rather than symptoms. Dr. Tom is also back practicing actively and seeing a near-normal patient load.

What message can we take home from Dr. Tom's experience? Perhaps that the body is a marvelously complex thing and that our efforts to understand it are only in their infancy. Dr. Tom's case shows the importance of looking at function rather than only disease or pathology. It shows the vital importance of investigating nutrition and metabolism. It illustrates how allopathic medicine and complementary medicine might merge their strengths to the ultimate benefit of the patient.

Laboratory Tests for the Difficult Case

There are numerous laboratory tests that are being used in the field of functional medicine that can help identify where your energy-producing process has gone awry. Each of us produces energy from our food in very predictable ways. The basic biochemistry is reasonably well understood. When someone suffers from fatigue it often suggests a disruption in the production of energy. It seems reasonable that to assess this we would run tests that look at the different energy pathways and the nutrients that drive them to determine where they are interrupted. These are precisely the kinds of tests that are becoming available. However, before describing these tests I want to point out some important myths about blood tests and other laboratory tests.

The Myth of the Lab Test: Function vs Pathology

Whenever you visit your doctor, the possibility exists that he or she will run some type of laboratory test, or blood test, to help determine what's wrong with you. Almost everyone has had the experience of going to the doctor with a problem, only to have the doctor say, "According to your lab tests, there isn't anything wrong with you," or "I have good news, your tests are normal, you're just fine." What accounts for the fact that our lab work is so often normal when, in fact, we are suffering terribly?

The answer may lie in two basic areas. First, many of the commonly ordered tests are only altered when disease or pathology exist. Second, the doctor must order the right tests to determine what's wrong. I'll explain a little about each of these areas.

The usual lab test you receive when you go to the doctor is called a SMAC and consists of 16-20 different tests such as serum cholesterol, bilirubin, liver enzymes called SGOT and SGPT, blood glucose, and so on. This test is a standard and provides a wealth of useful information. However, in most cases, these lab values aren't altered unless there is pathology, meaning that disease or destruction of cells must have already taken place. A good example of this are the liver enzymes SGOT and SGPT. When they are elevated, it usually means that some liver cells have been destroyed and the enzymes have leaked into the blood in greater amounts.

However, disease exists on a continuum. We are not healthy one day and diseased the next. There is usually a slow progression from excellent health to disease. Many lab tests only detect problems once they have reached the disease or pathologic state. The ideal tests would be those that measure changes in function as health is declining—before pathology exists.

Second, knowing which tests to order is part of the art and the science of medicine. If one does not ask the right question or look in the right area, one will not get the right answer. A perfect example is the case of an intelligent young girl who mysteriously began to develop mental retardation at age ten. Doctors ran test after test and had no clue as to what caused this drastic decline in her capability. One doctor finally suggested that they run a functional test. They looked at certain amino acid pathways in the body to see if they were working properly. Sure enough, her body was not converting certain amino acids, which suggested she was deficient in vitamin B_{12}. (The regular blood test for B_{12} had been normal.) After receiving injections for vitamin B_{12}, her health and mental function returned to normal.

We must remember that a blood test is like a snapshot. It often looks at what is happening in the body at the moment the blood is drawn and looks only at the items at which the doctor chooses to look. This is much like if you were on vacation taking photographs. Imagine you were busy taking pictures of the wildflowers on Mt. Ranier. Meanwhile, Bigfoot came running out of the forest behind you. You were occupied taking pictures of the flowers and were unaware of anything else going on around you. When later asked what you saw on the mountain, you would respond "wildflowers," when, in fact, Bigfoot was there. You missed it (perhaps the photo of the century). Likewise, the doctor who only orders a SMAC blood test on his fatigued patient might miss the fact that the patient has a deficiency of nutrients such as magnesium, tryptophan, taurine, tyrosine, B_1, B_6, and B_{12}. They are not a part of the snapshot.

Laboratory Tests

New laboratory tests are becoming available that allow us to look at functional changes before they lead to pathology. This is enabling doctors to see where changes in function are leading to symptoms and allowing doctors to specifically tailor treatment to the patient's individual biochemistry.

Below is a discussion of some of the tests and what you and your doctor can learn from them. Your present doctor may be unaware of these tests or how to interpret them. But the tests are performed by certified laboratories and are based on the most recent scientific research. Note that many of the tests are expensive. However, if your doctor is knowledgeable in biologic or functional medicine, he or she should be able to identify the tests that are most appropriate to your situation.

Amino acid analysis (blood or urine). Amino acids are the building blocks of protein in the body. They are components of proteins, enzymes, hormones, neurotransmitters, and other molecules. Amino acids are found in all food containing protein. When you eat chicken, beef, eggs, kidney beans, lima beans, and other protein-containing foods, the protein is broken down into a series of smaller molecules called amino acids. When amino acid function is disrupted, significant changes occur in energy metabolism, brain function, muscle function, heart function, and other processes that can lead to fatigue and many other adverse health consequences.

All amino acid metabolism is dependent upon adequate vitamins and minerals. If an amino acid, a key vitamin, or a key mineral is not present in sufficient amounts, the production of energy in the body can be disrupted. For example, vitamin B_6 is needed for almost all amino acid metabolism. If B_6 is deficient, amino acid metabolism is disrupted and energy production can be impaired.

Doctors who use amino acid analysis to determine their patients' state of health use urine or blood samples. Amino acid analysis from blood gives a better picture of which amino acids are deficient. Analysis from urine gives a better picture of which pathways are disrupted and which co-factors (vitamins, minerals) are deficient.

Recall the study I noted in chapter 4 in which Alexander Bralley, Ph.D., measured the amino acids of 25 patients with chronic fatigue syndrome. He and his colleagues found the most common deficiencies were (in order of frequency) tryptophan, phenylalanine, taurine, isoleucine, and leucine. The others were much less common. Bralley's group then supplemented each person with vitamin B_6, eight essential amino acids, and the amino acids that were deficient. After a three-month period of supplementation, near complete improvement in symptoms was seen in 75 percent of the people.[1]

Organic acid analysis. Organic acids is a term used to describe a large number of compounds derived from protein, fat, and carbohydrate. Organic acids are especially important in energy metabolism. For example, the Krebs cycle (or citric acid cycle) is one of the most important energy pathways in the body. One can now determine the status of Krebs cycle compounds including citrate, isocitrate, succinate, fumarate, malate, alpha-ketoglutarate, and cis-aconitate. This can shed light on where energy production might be blocked and gives insight into which vitamins, minerals, or amino acids might be needed therapeutically. Organic acid analysis is performed on urine.

Functional vitamin tests. When doctors take a blood sample to test for vitamins it is like a snapshot. It looks at only part of the scenery—blood serum. Most standard blood tests for vitamins do not take into consideration that there are other body substances or fluids that store vitamins and better reflect total body stores of a vitamin. B_{12} is a good example. Many cases have been reported of normal serum B_{12}, yet the patient improved on B_{12} supplements. Methylmalonic acid is a better test because it is a functional assessment. Some tests presently available for vitamins include the following.

- Thiamin (B_1): Erythrocyte transketolase (ETK)
- Riboflavin (B_2): Glutathione reductase (GSR)
- Cobalamin (B_{12}): Methylmalonic acid, amino acid analysis
- Niacin (B_3): 1-N-methylnicotinamide

- Folic acid: Homocysteine, formiminoglutamic acid
- Pyridoxine (B_6): Amino acid analysis, erythrocyte glutamate oxaloacetate transaminase (EGOT)
- Vitamin C: white blood cell ascorbate

Tests of Mineral Status

- Zinc: zinc loading test, red blood cell, whole blood, or hair. Zinc status is not easily assessed. More than one test is often used.
- Magnesium: red blood cell, magnesium loading test, or urine amino acids.
- Chromium: red blood cell, hair.
- Selenium: blood glutathione peroxidase, hair.
- Iron: serum ferritin, TIBC (total iron binding capacity).
- Calcium: ionized calcium, whole blood, 24-hour urine.
- Copper: red blood cell.
- Potassium: red blood cell.
- Manganese: red blood cell, hair, loading test.
- Molybdenum: serum uric acid, urine sulfite, hair.

Essential Fatty Acids. Essential fatty acids are needed for the formation of cell membranes, and they are used for fuel to produce energy to manufacture hormone-like substances called prostaglandins that influence inflammation and immune function. There are other uses for fatty acids as well. Tests for fatty acids can show whether deficiencies exist for certain fatty acids, whether certain co-factors are deficient, and whether certain pathways are blocked. This can form the basis for an appropriate supplementation program.

- Plasma fatty acid analysis
- Red cell fatty acid analysis
- Total lipid peroxides (shows damage to fatty acids and also reflects vitamin E status)
- Erythrocyte hemolysis. Shows how red blood cells withstand exposure to hydrogen peroxide. It is a crude indicator of vita-

min E status. This is important because vitamin E protects cell membrane fatty acids from damage by free radicals.

Functional Liver Detoxification Panel. The liver is one of the most complex organs in the body. It is here that the majority of environmental chemicals, additives, and microbial toxins are processed. Drugs and other toxins are also processed in the liver. Inadequate detoxication can result in a form of autointoxication, which can affect energy production. Tests being used to assess the detoxication pathways of the liver include:

- Salivary caffeine clearance
- Benzoate clearance
- Urinary sulfate/creatinine ratio

Tests for Dysbiosis (Microbial Overgrowth of Intestines)

It is now clear that the balance of helpful bacterial in the gut can be dramatically changed. Many factors can lead to the overgrowth of harmful bacteria, yeast, fungi, and parasites in the bowel. Each of these organisms release waste products that can be absorbed into the blood and can cause disruption of the body's energy system and many other systems. Modern laboratory techniques have allowed us to measure the specific chemicals (specific organic acids) given off by these microbes. The chemical substance identified in the urine helps to identify to some degree the kind of gut microbe causing trouble. An organic acid analysis that measures dysbiosis markers provides a window into the mystery of how the gut may influence mental and physical well being.

The substances typically measured include:

- p-hydroxybenzoate
- Tricarballylate
- Citramalate
- Tartarate
- p-hydroxyphenylacetate
- Dihydroxyphenylpropionate
- beta-keto-glutarate
- Arabinose

These tests can be extremely revealing. I recently measured the blood nutrient levels of a young man with fatigue, poor muscle strength, poor memory, concentration problems, and behavior difficulties. He was low in many important amino acids, fatty acids, vitamins, and minerals. Any time you see so many low nutrient values it is important to look for something that causes malabsorption of nutrients. In his case, the level of the chemical arabinose was extremely high in his urine. In fact, the upper limit of acceptable levels was less than 80. His was well above the reporting limits of the laboratory, which was 250. It was the highest level I have seen. His urine levels of dihydroxyphenylpropionate and p-hydroxyphenylacetate were also high.

Arabinose is a chemical produce by yeast such as Candida albicans. dihydroxyphenylpropionate is produced by bacteria called clostridia. Elevation of both of these is common with antibiotic overuse. Essentially, he had a severe intestinal infection that affected his nutrient absorption and, thus, his energy and health. Nutrient therapy along with biological agents to correct his dysbiosis has been very successful.

If you have chronic fatigue with any history of intestinal complaints, a dysbiosis panel like this looking for specific chemicals in urine is a vital step in unraveling the mystery of your chronic fatigue.

Tests for Toxicity

Chemical toxicity may be a contributor to chronic fatigue in some people. The tests below can help the doctor determine if toxic exposure has taken place, the extent of the damage, and if your detoxication processes are working properly.

- *Formic acid.* A test of how your body detoxifies formaldehyde and other aldehydes.
- *D-glucaric acid.* Measures if toxic exposure has taken place.
- *Mercapturic acid.* A metabolite of foreign chemicals and indicator of toxic exposure.
- *Total lipid peroxides.* Shows whether the lipids (or fats) that comprise your cell membranes are being damaged by free radicals.

- *Whole blood glutathione.* A compound in the body that binds to toxic chemicals to facilitate their elimination.

- *Glutathione peroxidase.* A compound that helps protect cells from free-radical damage, and stimulates glutathione to bind to chemical toxins.

- *Amino acid analysis.* Assesses many aspects of metabolism and function. Shows amino acid deficiencies, and vitamin and mineral deficiencies.

- *Serum and red blood cell vitamins and minerals.* Identifies the status of nutrients needed in detoxication of chemicals.

- *Provocation-neutralization test.* Done in a physician's office, this test determines sensitivity to chemicals and identifies a neutralizing dose that can be helpful in reducing symptoms.

- *Blood and urine tests for pesticides and industrial chemicals.*

A beginning laboratory panel that one might consider to assess toxicity might include:[5]

Mercapturic acid	D-glucaric acid
Formic acid	Glutathione peroxidase
Lipid peroxides	

Toxic Minerals. Toxic minerals such as lead, mercury, cadmium, aluminum, arsenic, and nickel all have the capacity to induce fatigue. Measurement of these metals can be done on urine, hair, or blood.

- Hair analysis is considered an useful screening test. It is inexpensive and easily obtained.

- Urine analysis after a challenge with EDTA, DMSA, DMPS, or penicillamine is also useful.

- Red cell analysis for toxic metals is also used.

- MELISA. Measures immune cell reactivity to toxic minerals.

Tests of Antioxidant Status and Oxidant Stress. Our bodies are constantly producing highly reactive free radicals as a part of the normal detoxication pathways and immune defenses. Our normal system of protection that ensures our tissues will not be destroyed by the free radicals encompasses the antioxidant nutrients (vitamins C and E, beta-carotene, lycopene, glutathione, coenzyme Q, etc.) and the antioxidant enzymes (mineral-dependent). If the free-radical load becomes too great, if antioxidant stores are too low, or if a combination of the two occurs, free-radical damage can occur. A test is now available that looks at oxidant and antioxidant status and has been a useful tool for doctors who work with a variety of chronic health complaints.

- Thiobarbituric acid-reactive substances.
- Pantox panel including:

Coenzyme Q_{10} (ubiquinol)	Alpha-tocopherol (vitamin E)
Gamma-tocopherol	Lycopene
Beta-carotene	Alpha-carotene
Vitamin A	Ascorbic acid
Uric acid	Bilirubin

- Whole blood glutathione
- Iron status. Iron is a pro-oxidant.

Tests for Immunologic Function. Many cases of chronic fatigue are associated with immune system abnormalities. Included might be immune deficiency, immune hyperreactivity, or problems with immune repair. Assessment of immune function is a rapidly growing science, but not all immune measurements give a clear indication of what is wrong. Certain assessments of immune status can, in fact, give conflicting results. Nevertheless, certain tests can be helpful. These include:

- Natural killer cells
- T-helper cells
- T-suppressor cells
- Helper/suppressor ratio
- Erythrocyte sedimentation rate (ESR).

- CBC with differential white count.
- Salivary IgA. Measures the primary antibody produced in the mouth and intestinal tract that is directed against viral invaders.
- IgG food and environmental panel

A Complex Field

In this chapter, I have described a number of tests that might be helpful in understanding certain metabolic factors that contribute to fatigue. Please realize that there are many other tests available that provide further insights into the functioning of the body. The discussion above is merely a general introduction to a very complex field of study.

Chapter 28

Questions You Might Ask

ONE OF THE MOST valuable things you can do in determining the origin of your fatigue is to look carefully at your personal history and ask a series of questions. These questions can be extremely helpful in your quest for solutions and can also help your doctor better understand the mysteries of your illness. Remember, many doctors are overbooked, running behind schedule, and pressured under the confines of a five-, ten-, or fifteen-minute office call. It simply is not enough time to do an adequate history and examination of a patient with chronic fatigue. Therefore, the more information you can provide about key associations you have uncovered, the better. We will look at a number of important questions and discuss their implications below.

1. Was the onset sudden or slow? Is there a periodicity to the "fatigue" cycle? If the onset was sudden, was it associated with the flu, mononucleosis, or other infection?

2. Is this the first or is this a repeated experience? If recurrent, how does this event compare/contrast with other similar events?

3. Were there any specific events prior to the initial onset that are of note?

A. Exposure to new living or working environments? Bill A. developed his fatigue after moving into a new home. Similarly, workers at the EPA (Environmental Protection Agency) became sick and had to leave work after moving into their new headquarters.

B. Travel (exhaustion, diarrhea, medications, chemical exposures . . .). If you return from a trip to Mexico or Asia with diarrhea, it is possible that you contracted an intestinal parasite. Your doctor should thoroughly investigate that possibility. Exhaustion and exposure are very common on trips as well. As a Midwesterner who travels extensively, I've watched many a tourist be overcome by the combination of rich food, lack of sleep, excessive sun exposure, wind, alcohol, breakneck pacing, and other factors of travel that simply wear them out. Exhaustion sets in and they feel lousy. Usually this passes, but in some people it can be a trigger.

C. Are others affected by the same condition? If your entire family is effected by sickness and symptoms of fatigue you may need to look for a common exposure to parasites, chemicals, or otherwise. The culprit may be in your home. Bill A., whom I mentioned earlier, became sick after moving into a new home. His wife and six-year-old daughter also developed significant respiratory problems. I knew we were really on to something when I discovered their dog had developed a bad cough and labored breathing after moving into the new home. The home was later found to have been sprayed with chlordane, a termiticide. As we've seen, chemical exposure is an important contributor to fatigue.

Ask your co-workers if they've developed any unusual symptoms lately or if they are fatigued. You and your doctor could spend a lot of time barking up the wrong tree if you neglect to ask this question and it turns out half the office staff has been feeling sluggish because of the remodeling next door. Chemicals are used extensively in office buildings, schools, nursing homes, hospitals, and elsewhere. Remodeling of office buildings goes on constantly, which often includes the use of glues and adhesives, varnish and stain, new carpet or vinyl floor covering, and an endless list of synthetic material. Recall the Washington, D.C. home for the elderly, in which 350 volatile organic chemicals were found circulating in the indoor air.

D. Smoke or fire exposure? Pollutant molecules, gases, and vapors can linger if not properly dealt with. Fire departments often use ozone generators to remove some of the vapors, but you must never be in the home when this is done.

E. Starting or stopping medications? Fatigue is a major or minor side effect of a substantial number of prescription drugs. Moreover, if you are taking more than one drug the likelihood of interactive side effects increases. If you have recently started, stopped, or changed a medication, look seriously at whether the drug may be a factor. Asking this simple question could save you a lot of time and anxiety as you search for the cause of your fatigue.

F. Relationship change? Have you recently fallen in love, or perhaps broken up with someone with whom you were serious?

G. Family structure change? Have you been involved in a divorce, separation, or custody battle? Have you lost a family member to accident or illness? Do you live with a spouse, parent, or child who is chemically dependent? Do you live with a spouse or parent who is abusive? Have you remarried? Have you adopted children, added children through birth, or added children through remarriage?

H. Job satisfaction and occupational toxicant exposures? Job dissatisfaction is a major source of stress in industrialized cultures, and excessive stress is a major source of fatigue and illness. Look carefully at your work situation.

Also, chemical exposure on the job can contribute to fatigue. David H. was a professional painter of homes and offices. He was fatigued much of the day and evening. When I asked him whether the paint and varnish fumes ever bothered him he said "no," but then added, "Some days when I get home I'm so exhausted I fall to the couch and the room just sort of spins around." Paula D. was a professional sign painter who suffered from fatigue and migraine headaches. She was found (by hair mineral analysis) to have high lead and cadmium in her body. Lead, cadmium, and other heavy metals contribute to fatigue by a variety of means. I've also worked with many chemists who became ill and fatigued because of their exposure to chemicals at work.

I. Sexual history (sexually transmitted diseases such as chlamydia, Herpes, Papilloma virus, gonorrhea, HIV, syphilis, candida)? Also look at sexual preferences, libido, sexual ease, etc. People with a history of sexually transmitted disease often have a history of antibiotic overuse—another contributor to fatigue.

J. Pregnancy? Fatigue is common during pregnancy and certainly common in the postpartum period. Bearing and raising any child can be challenging, but twins or triplets can be demanding both physically and emotionally. If births are closely spaced, this also can be nutritionally and emotionally very demanding. For example, I've commonly heard from patients (and this has be corroborated by doctors to whom I lecture), "I've never been the same since my second child," or "I was really never ill until after my second child." I've observed this to be true especially if the children were born nine to eighteen months apart. So if you are a parent with two or three or four kids under the age of five, your fatigue may be due to circumstances. Parents of children of any age fit this bill.

4. Do you have a family history of chronic allergies, endocrine dysfunction, depression? If your parents had allergies, there is a good chance you may also suffer from allergy. If a parent suffered from thyroid problems—which can run in families—you may need to be evaluated for thyroid dysfunction.

5. Were you a "difficult child" with history of colic or GI distress? This may reflect nutritional problems or exposure. Recall that gastrointestinal problems are associated with fatigue for many different reasons.

6. Were you breastfed as a child? If so, what was your mother's health at the time? When was the previous pregnancy? Studies of African tribes conducted by Dr. Weston Price found that children born soon after a previous child tended to suffer more health problems. This was presumably because the nutritional demands of the previous birth deprived the subsequent child of needed nutrients.

7. Are you adversely affected by any smells, aromas, or volatile chemicals? This is an indication that you may have multiple chemical sensitivity, which suggests widespread nutritional deficiency.

Also, people with yeast-related illness suffer from sensitivity to odors. Likewise, those with immune system problems, either underactive or overactive, may suffer this way.

8. Are you exposed to and affected by molds? Mold sensitivity can contribute to mild to extreme fatigue. If you are unable to identify the origins of your fatigue it is worth having a blood test to assess your sensitivity to mold. One way in which mold contributes to fatigue is by contributing to chronically congested sinuses. There are many other means such as through chronic immune activation.

9. What links have you made between your condition, and what improves or worsens your state of health? Be sure to give this information to your doctor. Doctors are taught to value this information, but not all doctors do.

10. Have there been recent changes in diet, and is diet balanced for your individual needs? Have you changed your diet in dramatic ways? I've observed many patients who, after beginning a weight loss program, become fatigued. In many of these cases, the program was too low in calories and too low in protein, so the patient began to metabolize their own muscle tissue. If you're on a weight-loss program, check with a nutrition-oriented health professional to see if it is adequate. I've also observed cases in which the patient has begun to consume excessive calories and becomes sluggish or tired. This is common in winter months when people sit a lot, eat a lot, and don't get any sun.

Some people who switch to a vegetarian or macrobiotic diet become fatigued. These diets are generally very helpful if properly balanced for protein and other nutrients. Deficiency of vitamin B_{12} can become significant in vegetarians. Vitamin B_{12} deficiency can lead to substantial fatigue. Carnitine insufficiency may also occur in vegetarians.

11. What symptom patterns provide clues? Do these occur in relation to specific hours, days, situations, or events? Observe for patterns in your symptoms. If you are fatigued only on weekdays and feel good or great on weekends, think about job stress, job dissatisfaction, co-worker conflicts, or other work-related aspects. Also think

about chemical exposure on the job, or indoor air pollutants at the office or plant. If you feel great during the week but fatigued on weekends, it may be related to overwork where you just collapse on your days off. It may also be related to family stress at home or perhaps pollutant exposure at home.

12. Is there anyone else who has the same or similar situation? Again, look at your family members and co-workers. If they also suffer from symptoms you have an important clue. Also, question your friends with whom you recently traveled to Guatemala. You all may have picked up a "bug" of some sort.

Food-borne infection is a growing problem in the United States and other industrialized countries. If you become sick or fatigued following a meal, either at home or at a restaurant, check with your dining partners to see if they suffered similarly.

13. Do you believe it is possible to get better? If not, why not? If you have suffered from fatigue for months or years and doctor after doctor has been unable to help you, a bit of frustration or even cynicism is understandable. However, if you don't believe it is possible to get better, it may reflect an aspect of your personality or viewpoint that actually impairs immunity, and thus your potential for recovery. For example, optimists have more active immune systems than pessimists. Pessimists suffer more infections and more illness than optimists. A pessimistic outlook can be a self-fulfilling prophecy. Fortunately, so can an optimistic outlook.

14. Maternal and paternal nutrition/alcoholism? Chronic alcohol consumption can contribute to serious nutritional problems and fatigue. Living with an alcoholic family member can be enormously stressful.

15. Childhood diet: 'empty calories,' dietary eccentricities, pica? If your childhood diet was poor, chances are good that many of the habits continued into adulthood. Nutrient deficiencies may have developed. You food choices may be directly contributing to your fatigue. In these instances, dietary improvements often help substantially.

16. History of abuse or neglect? Researchers at the University of Medicine and Dentistry of New Jersey assessed the effects of childhood abuse on the rate of illness in women. Fifty-three percent of the women reported suffering one or more kinds of abuse (physical, emotional, or sexual) as children. The women reporting abuse were more likely to report symptoms of fatigue, insomnia, and headaches.[1]

17. Antibiotic therapy history? Several recent studies have linked the overuse of antibiotics with development of chronic fatigue and other chronic complaints.

18. What is your level of physical activity? Sedentary people often have less active immune systems and also fatigue more easily. In contrast, athletes who overtrain may suffer from fatigue for various reasons.[2] (Questions reprinted with permission Intl Clin Nutr Rev.)

Is This the Right Doctor for You?
Questions to Ask Your Doctor

Now that you've asked yourself the questions about fatigue, it is time to find a doctor with whom you can work. There are a couple of reasons for this discussion. Many doctors do not like to work with patients whose main complaint is chronic fatigue. To them it is a diagnostic quagmire with few road signs. It takes up a lot of their time. Moreover, their rate of success might be low, making treatment of these patients somewhat unrewarding. It can be a complicated mess that many doctors would rather avoid. So a few questions you may wish to ask the doctor or staff over the phone are:

1. Do you work with patients who have chronic fatigue?
2. Do you like to work with patients who have chronic fatigue?
3. Do you have a system for diagnosis and treatment of patients with chronic fatigue?
4. What is your rate of success with fatigued patients?
5. Do you consider the nutritional needs of your fatigued patients?

The doctor who does not work with or who does not like to work with fatigued patients may not be the right one for you. The doctor who does not have a strategy, method, or system for diagnosis and treatment of fatigued patients may not quickly and efficiently identify the source of your problem. Remember, chronic fatigue can be a very complicated disorder. Not all doctors are familiar with the spectrum of factors that must be considered. This is *especially* true of the nutritional, environmental, and allergic factors.

Once you get in the doctors office, you want to determine whether or not he or she is one with whom you can work. It is important that your personal philosophy of how you would like to be treated is compatible with theirs. The chances for success are much greater if this is so. Below is a list of questions that you may wish to ask your prospective doctor in this regard.

1. Would you be comfortable with my asking you about ten questions so I can better understand your care of me? (If the doctor is uncomfortable, stop and consider seeking another doctor.)

2. Do you expect to tell me what to do, or to explain my options and let me choose?

3. How much time will we have at each visit to answer my questions?

4. Do you welcome me as a participant in my care?

5. Do you think I can understand my conditions and play an active role in my care?

6. What preventive measures do you advocate so I can avoid getting sick?

7. Do you keep a list of all my medicines to minimize the chance of adverse interactions?

8. Are you aware of the potential adverse or beneficial effects of the environment on me?

9. How do you stay up on all the advances made in medicine?

10. How would you explain to me bad news, if it were ever necessary?

If you feel awkward asking these questions, let the doctor know. If the doctor expresses awkwardness in answering, thank them for their humanity and candor. You deserve the best possible care and the above questions can help you select the best possible doctor available.[3]

Epilogue

IN WRITING THIS BOOK, I have attempted to cover the topic of chronic fatigue in as broad a manner as possible, while still maintaining a book of readable length. In such an undertaking, one invariably leaves important elements out of the discussion. This is certainly the case with chronic fatigue. Two topics deserving of discussion are traditional Chinese Medicine and homeopathy. Both systems of medicine are comprehensive in their approach, and are unique in their philosophy and methodology.

Homeopathy developed over 200 years ago when Dr. Samuel Hahnemann discovered that substances causing one set of symptoms in concentrated doses, could remedy those same symptoms when given in microdoses. He also discovered that the more a remedy is diluted, the greater its potency. This system evolved over many years into a complex medical system that is gaining increasing acceptance worldwide. In fact, the World Health Organization has cited homeopathy as one of the systems of traditional medicine that should be integrated worldwide with conventional medicine in order to provide adequate global health care by the year 2000.

Homeopathic medicine can be extremely effective in both curing and relieving symptoms of chronic fatigue. This is an important distinction. Some people have found success using combination remedies to improve their energy. This is different from one in which a homeopathic practitioner takes a careful history and prescribes a remedy to affect the fundamental nature of the illness. In my opinion, homeopathic medicine is a wise choice in the overall care of illness. This is certainly true of chronic fatigue.*

---

*For more information see *Discovering Homeopathy: Your Introduction to*

Traditional Chinese medicine has evolved over several thousand years. It is generally described as including acupuncture, food or diet therapy, herbal medicine, movement therapy such as *t'ai chi,* energy work such as *chi kung,* and massage. The treatments in traditional Chinese Medicine are very specific to the individual depending on their pattern of disharmony. In traditional Chinese Medicine, chronic fatigue may be due to a number of different patterns. Practitioners of traditional Chinese Medicine have success in treating chronic fatigue because their treatment is directed at the specific pattern, regardless of its apparent origin. In this way, traditional Chinese Medicine can help remedy fatigue that is due to liver disorders, psychological imbalance, seasonal factors, reproductive problems, immune abnormalities, and even constitutional factors. It is impossible to even attempt to describe, in this short discussion, the elaborate system that is traditional Chinese Medicine. My point is to suggest that traditional Chinese Medicine offers a solution to chronic fatigue sufferers that is as valid and useful as that which is described in this book.** The method is very different, but the result may be the same.

I have attempted to convey in this book the need for wholeness and balance. Systems such as traditional Chinese Medicine and homeopathy are among those that treat the patient as a whole and unique being. We must recognize that the current model of medicine based on an arbitrary separation of the different systems of the human body does not serve us. One can convincingly argue that the body is not separate from the soul, the mind is not separate from the body, the human is not separate from the environment, and that an individual, while unique in many ways, is not separate from other individuals. The individual is a part of the dynamic interaction between all of these systems, and is not free of interdependence. Our present medical model has separated these systems for convenience

---

the Science and Art of Homeopathic Medicine, by Dana Ullman (North Atlantic Books, Berkeley, California 1991).

**For more information see *Between Heaven and Earth: A Guide to Chinese Medicine,* by H. Beinfeld and E. Korngold.

and to fully understand them, but separate from interaction with co-dependent systems, they stand artificially alone.

Many ancient methods of healing have recognized the dynamic interrelationship between all things. They possess a unique wisdom and insight. As medicine moves forward, it will always simultaneously enfold the rich heritage of the past. As we begin to weave the fabric of the past, present, and future we will hopefully come closer to understanding who we are. In this journey, we will likely be humbled by the awesome power, beauty, complexity, and simplicity of the body's ability to heal itself with more than mechanical tinkering from ourselves.

Appendix A

Laboratory Services for Assessment of Nutrient Status, Immune Function, and Toxicity

BELOW IS A directory of laboratories that provide specialized diagnostic services. These are labs that offer most of the tests described in this book. Most labs also have a list of health care professionals who use their services. In this way, a lab may be able to help you locate a doctor who is familiar with a particular form of assessment.

Laboratory	*Service*
Accu-Chem Laboratories 990 North Bowser Road Suite 800 Richardson, TX 75081	Toxics such as pesticides, etc. (in blood and urine)
Pacific Toxicology 1545 Pontius Avenue Los Angeles, California 90025	Toxic substances in blood and urine
Serammune Physicians Laboratory 1890 Preston White Drive Reston, Virginia 22091	Delayed immune reaction to food, environmental, and chemical substances
Immuno Laboratories 1620 West Oakland Pk. Blvd. Fort Lauderdale, Florida 33311	Delayed immune reaction (IgG) to food; candida antibody, EBV antibody

Diagnos-Techs, Inc.
6620 S. 192nd Place, J-104
Kent, Washington 98032

Salivary cortisol and DHEA

Great Smokies Diagnostic Laboratory
63 Zillicoa St.
Asheville, North Carolina 28801

Stool analysis, parasitology, intestinal permeability measure, secretory IgA, breath gases, liver function/detoxication

MetaMetrix Medical Laboratory
500 Peachtree Industrial Blvd.
Norcross, Georgia 30071

Amino acids, organic acids, intestinal permeability, fatty acids

Meridian Valley Clinical Lab
24030 132nd Avenue S.E.
Kent, Washington 98042

Stool analysis, detoxification, secretory IgA, adrenal profile, blood or urine amino acids

Doctor's Data, Inc.
P.O. Box 111
West Chicago, Illinois 60185

Amino acids, hair mineral, red cell toxic minerals, whole blood trace elements, D-glucaric acid, mercapturic acid, urine toxic minerals

Monroe Medical Laboratory
Route 17, P.O. Box 1
Southfield, New York 10975

Vitamins, minerals, essential fatty acids, etc.

Pantox Laboratories
4622 Santa Fe Street
San Diego, California 92109

Serum antioxidants including vitamin A, E, C, ß-carotene, coenzyme Q10, lycopene, iron and lipid status

SpectraCell Laboratories
515 Post Oak Blvd., Suite 830
Houston, Texas 77027

Lymphocyte analysis for 19 nutrients including B-vitamins, some minerals, and some amino acids, oxidative stress profile

Immunodiagnostics
488 McCormick St.
San Leandro, California 94577

Immune system parameters

Appendix B

Our Mission

Our mission is to create the opportunity for wholeness of body, mind, and spirit within individuals and society. We believe that within each person lies the spark of love and creativity that, if given the chance to germinate, brings richness to life.

In recognition that the journey for many people is met with economic difficulty we have dedicated a portion of the proceeds from all of our books and professional efforts to provide:

1. Free health care to families with great need
2. Free nutritional products to children and families who lack the resources

While we currently provide free counsel to many, it is our hope that one day we may support a clinic where all can receive care without charge.

Michael A. Schmidt
Julie A. Schmidt

References

Chapter 1: The Many Faces of Fatigue

1. Grierson, H, Holmes, GP, Straus, SE. Coping with chronic fatigue syndrome. Patient Care 1987 (Nov. 15):79–82.

2. *Fibromyalgia Network, New CFS criteria 1994: October: 6, p. 6).* The covference was the 17th International Symposium on Repetitive Stree Injuries, Fibromalgyia, and Chronic Fatigue Syndrome sponsored by the Physical Medicine and Rehabilitation Foundation, Vancouver, B.B., October, 1994.

Chapter 2: Intestinal Problems

1. Intestinal Permeability: In Application Guide (Asheville, North Carolina: Great Smokies Diagnostic Laboratory, 1992).

2. Anonymous. How does IP apply to AIDS patients and those suffering from chronic fatigue? Smokies Digest 1993 (June–August):7.

3. Shrive, E, et al. Glutamine in treatment of peptic ulcer. Tex J Med 1957; 53:840–843.

4. Kimberg, V, et al. Oral glutamine accelerates the healing of the small intestine and improves outcome after whole abdominal radiation. Arch Surg 1990; 15:1040–1045.

5. Ackerson, A, Resnick, C. The effects of L-glutamine, N-acetyl-D-Glucosamine, gamma-linolenic acid and gamma-oryzanol on intestinal permeability. Townsend Letter Doctors 1993 (Jan):20–23.

6. Burton, AF, et al. Decreased incorporation of 14C-Glusamine relative to 3H-N-Acetyl glucosamine in the intestinal mucosa of patients with inflammatory bowel disease. Am J Gastro Ent 1983; 78 (1):19–22.

7. Petschow, BW, Talbott, RD. Response of bifidobacterium species to growth promoters in human and cow milk. Pediatric Res 1991; 29 (2):208–13.

8. Ghannoum, MA, et al. Protection against Candida albicans gastrointestinal colonization and dissemination by saccharides in experimental animals. Microbios 1991; 67 (271):95–105.

9. Hunter, JO, Jones, VA. Food and the Gut (Philadelphia: Balliere Tindal, 1985).

10. Bentley, SJ, Pearson, DJ, Rix, KJB. Food hypersensitivity in irritable bowel syndrome. Lancet 1983 (Aug. 6):295–297.

11. Petitpierre, M, Gumowski, P, Girard, JP. Irritable bowel syndrome and hypersensitivity to food. Ann Allergy 1985; 54:538–49.

12. Zwethckenbaum, J, Burakoff, R. Irritable bowel syndrome and food hypersensitivity. Ann Allergy 1988; 61:47–49.

13. Fell, PJ, Soulby, S, Brostoff, J. Cellular responses to food in irritable bowel syndrome—an investigation of the ALCAT test. J Nutr Med 1991; 2:143–49.

14. Galland, L, Lee, M. High-frequency giardiasis in patients with chronic digestive complaints. (Abstract) Am J Gastroenterol 1989; 84:1181.

15. Jaffe, RM. Nutritional Immunology: 1992–1993 Syllabus (Reston, Virginia: Health Studies Collegium, 1992).

16. Bland, JS. Management of irritable bowel syndrome. In Advancement in Clinical Nutrition (Gig Harbor, Washington: HealthComm, 1994)2–15.

Chapter 3: Food and Fatigue

1. Speer, F (ed). Allergy of the Nervous System (Springfield, Illinois: Charles C. Thomas, 1970).

2. Randolph, T. The Alternative Approach to Allergies (New York: Lippincott & Crowell, 1979):138–140.

3. Philpott, W. Brain Allergies (New Canaan, Connecticut: Keats Publishing, 1981).

4. USDA (United States Department of Agriculture): Economic Research Service, Sugar and Sweeteners. Situation and Outlook report yearbook. (Washington, D.C.: U.S. Government Printing Office, 1989):81.

5. Smith, R. Organic foods vs. supermarket foods: element levels. J Appl Nutr 1993; 45 (1):35–39.

6. Mott, L, Snyder, K. Pesticide Alert: a Guide to Pesticides in Fruits and Vegetables (New York: NRDC, 1987):23.

7. Walton, RG, Hudak, R, Green-Waite, RJ. Adverse reactions to aspartame: Double-blind challenge in patients from a vulnerable population. Biol Psych 1993; 34:13–17.

8. Wurtman, J. Managing Your Mind & Mood Through Food (New York: Harper & Row, 1988):17–31.

9. Spring, B, et al. Psychobiological effects of carbohydrates. J Clin Psychiatry 1989; 50 (Suppl):27–33.

10.Wurtman, J. Managing Your Mind & Mood Through Food (New York: Harper & Row, 1988):26.

11. Ibid.

Chapter 4: Vitamins, Minerals, and Fatigue

1. Blumberg, J. Assessing immunological function across the lifespan. International Symposium on Functional Medicine, Maui, Hawaii, 1993.

2. Hume, P, Wyers, E. Changes in leukocyte ascorbic acid during the common cold. Scottish Med J 1973; 18:3–7.

3. Pangborn, J. Personal communication, 1993.

4. Cheney, PR. Chronic fatigue syndrome as a metabolic disorder. CFIDS Chronicle 1993 (Summer):1–6.

5. Bralley, JA. Personal communication, 1993.

6. Pangborn, J. Functional amino acid abnormalities. Personal communication, 1993.

7. Kuratsune, H, et al. Acylcarnitine deficiency in chronic fatigue syndrome. Clin Infect Dis 1994; 18 (suppl 1):S62–S67.

8. Reichmann, H, Lindeneiner, N. Carnitine analysis in normal human red blood cells, plasma, and muscle tissue. European Neurology 1994; 34:40–43.

9. Lapp, CW, Cheney, PR. Chronic Fatigue Self-Care Manual, 1991.

10. Bliznakov, EG. Miracle Nutrient: Coenzyme Q10 (New York: Bantam, 1987).

11. Behan, PO, Behan, WMH, Horrobin, DF. Placebo-controlled trial of n-3 and n-6 essential fatty acids in the treatment of post-viral fatigue syndrome. Acta Neurologica Scandinavica 1990; 82:209–16.

12. Schmidt, MA. Childhood Ear Infections (Berkeley, California: North Atlantic Books, 1990):96.

13. Trans fatty acids in foods. Nutr Rev 1984:42 (8).

14. Enig, MG, Pallansch, LA, Sampugna, J, Keeney, M. Fatty acid composition of the fat in selected food items with emphasis on trans components. J Am Oil Chem Soc 1983; 60:1788–95.

15. Subar, AF, et al. Folate intake and food sources in the US population. Am J Clin Nutr 1989; 50:508–16.

16. Rea, W. Chemical Sensitivity (Boca Raton, Florida: Lewis Publishers, 1993):263.

17. Schneider, D, et al. Blood glutathione: a biochemical index of aging women. Fed Proc Am Soc Exp Biol 1982; 41:3570.

18. Waryshkin, S, et al. Blood glutathione: a biochemical index of human aging. Fed Proc Am Soc Exp Biol 1981; 40:3179.

19. Kilburn, KH, et al. Neurobehavioral dysfunction in firemen exposed to polychlorinated biphenyls (PCBs): possible improvement after detoxification. Arch Env Hlth 1989; 44:345–50.

20. Cox, IM, Campbell, MJ, Dowson, D. Red blood cell magnesium and chronic fatigue syndrome. Lancet 1991; 337:757–60.

21. Crook, WG. Chronic Fatigue Syndrome and the Yeast Connection (Jackson, Tennessee: Professional Books 1993):252.

22. Ibid, 253.

23. Seelig, M, Cantin, M. (eds) Magnesium in Health and Disease: Proceedings of the 2nd International Symposium on Magnesium (New York: Spectrum Books, 1980).

24. Rogers, SA. Unrecognized magnesium deficiency masquerades as diverse symptoms: evaluation of an oral magnesium challenge test. Intl Clin Nutr Rev 1991; 11 (3):117–29.

25. Wester, P. Magnesium. Am J Clin Nutr 1987; 45:1305–12.

26. Franz, KB. Magnesium intake during pregnancy. Magnesium 1987; 6:18–27.

27. Rea, W. Chemical Sensitivity (Boca Raton, Florida: Lewis Publishers, 1993):307.

28. Baker, S. Magnesium chloride as a therapeutic agent. Personal communication, 1994.

29. Rajagopalan, KV. Molybdenum: an essential trace element in human nutrition. Ann Rev Nutr 1988; 8:400–427.

30. Pangborn, JB. Minerals: Clinical and Physiological Significance (Chicago, Illinois: Bionostics, Inc., 1993):8.

31. Fox, HM. J Nutr Sci Vitaminol (Tokyo), August, 1976.

32. Podell, RN. Doctor, Why Am I So Tired? (New York: Pharos Books, 1987):41. Dr. Lonsdale's work is briefly reviewed.

33. Eisinger, J, Zakarian, H, Plantamura, A, Clairet, D, Ayavou, T. Studies of transketolase in chronic pain. J Adv Med 1992; 5 (2):105–113.

34. Finglas, PM. Thiamin. Flair Concerted Action 1994; 10:270–273.

35. Kant, AK, Block, G. Dietary vitamin B$_6$ intake and food sources in

the US population: NHANES II, 1976–1980. Am J Clin Nutr 1990; 52:707–16.

36. Rea, W. Chemical Sensitivity (Boca Raton, Florida: Lewis Publishers, 1993):256.

37. Manore, MM, et al. Plasma pyridoxal-5-phosphate concentration and dietary B6 intake in free-living, low-income elderly people. Am J Clin Nutr 1989; 50:339–45.

38. Heller, S, et al. Vitamin B6 status in pregnancy. Am J Clin Nutr 1973; 26 (12):1339–48.

39. Br Med J 1956; 2:1394–1399.

40. N Engl J Med 1988; 318:1720–28.

41. Br J Nutr 1973; 30:277–83

42. Bralley, JA. Personal communication, 1993.

43. Jaffe, RM. The great B12 robbery. In Nutritional Immunology: 1992–1993 Syllabus (Reston, Virginia: Health Studies Collegium, 1992).

44. Lederle, FA. Oral cobalamine for pernicious anemia: Medicine's best kept secret? JAMA 1991; 265 (1):94–95.

45. Cheraskin, E. Daily vitamin C consumption and fatigability. J Am Ger Soc 1976:24 (3); 136–37.

46. Maiani, G, et al. Vitamin C. Flair Concerted Action #10 Status Papers, 1994; 289–295.

47. Rogers, S. Tired or Toxic? (Syracuse, New York: Prestige Publishers, 1990):152–53.

48. Crook, WG. Chronic Fatigue Syndrome and the Yeast Connection (Jackson, Tennessee: Professional Books, 1993):252.

49. Holden, JM, et al. Zinc and copper in self-selected diets. J Am Diet Assoc 1979; 75:23.

50. Bogden, JD, et al. Zinc and immunocompetence in the elderly: Baseline data on zinc nutriture and immunity in unsupplemented subjects. Am J Clin Nutr 1987; 46 (1):101–109.

Chapter 5: Blood Sugar Disorders

1. Gaby, AR, Wright, JV. Nutritional regulation of blood glucose. J Adv Med 1991; 4 (1):57–71.

2. USDA (United States Department of Agriculture): Economic Research Service, Sugar and Sweeteners. Situation and Outlook report yearbook. (Washington, D.C.: U.S. Government Printing Office, 1989):81.

3. Karjalainen, J, et al. A bovine albumin peptide as a possible trigger of insulin-dependent diabetes mellitus. N Engl J Med 1992; 327:302–307.

4. Hambridge, KM, Rogerson, DD, O'Brien, D. Concentration of chromium in the hair of normal children and children with juvenile diabetes mellitus. Diabetes 1968; 17 (8):517–518.

5. Boyle, E, et al. Chromium depletion in the pathogenesis of diabetes and atherosclerosis. S Med J 1977; 70 (12):1449–1453.

6. Kozlovsky, AS, et al. Effects of diets high in simple sugars on urinary chromium losses. Metabolism 1986; 35:515.

7. Rohn, J, et al. Magnesium, zinc and copper in plasma and blood cellular components in children with insulin-dependent diabetes mellitus. Clin Chem A 1993; 215:21–28.

8. Araki, A, et al. Plasma homocysteine concentrations in Japanese patients with non-insulin-dependent diabetes mellitus: Effect of parenteral methylcobalamin treatment. Atherosclerosis 1993; 103:149–57.

9. Pecoraro, RE, Chen, MS. Ascorbic acid metabolism in diabetes mellitus. In Third Conference on Vitamin C. Ann NY Acad Sci 1987:498.

10. Goodman, S. Vitamin C: The Master Nutrient (New Canaan, Connecticut: Keats Publishing, Inc. 1991):60.

11. Gaby, AR, Wright, JV. Nutritional regulation of blood glucose. J Adv Med 1991; 4 (1):57–71.

12. Breneman, JC. Basics of Food Allergy (Springfield, Illinois: Charles C. Thomas, 1978).

13. Effects of exercise on insulin sensitivity in humans. Diabetes Care 1992; 15 (Suppl 4):1690.

Chapter 6: Elevated Blood Fats

1. Willett, WC, Ascherio, A. Trans fatty acids: Are the effects only marginal? Am J Pub Hlth 1994; 84 (5):722–724.

Chapter 7: Overweight and Underlean

1. Newberne, PM. Overnutrition in resistance of dogs to distemper virus. Fedn Proc 1966; 25:1701–1710.

2. Bland, JS, Dibiase, F, Ronzio, R. Physiological effects of a doctor-supervised versus an unsupervised over-the-counter weight loss program. J Nutr Med 1992; 3:285–293.

3. Anonymous. Weight loss without dietary restriction: Efficacy of different forms of aerobic exercise. Am J Sports Med 1987; 15 (3):275.

4. Anonymous. The effect of weight loss by dieting or exercise on resting metabolic rate in overweight men. Int J Obesity 1990; 14:327.

5. Anonymous. Prostaglandins, brown fat, and weight loss. Med Hypoth 1989; 28:13.

Chapter 8: Thyroid and Adrenal Trouble

1. Langer. S. Solved: The Riddle of Illness (New Canaan, Connecticut: Keats Publishing, 1984):24–32.

2. van Raaji, JAGM, et al. Neurotoxic chlorinated hydrocarbons penetrate the blood-brain barrier possibly by binding to thyroid hormone transport proteins. Neurotoxicology 1991; 12 (4):818.

3. Carter-Pokras, O, Brody, D, Murphy, RS. Selected pesticide residues and metabolites in urine from a survey of the U.S. general population. J Tox Env Hlth 1992; 37:277–291.

4. Sehnert, K. Personal communication, 1994.

5. Podell, RN. Doctor, Why Am I So Tired? (New York: Pharos Books, 1987):151.

6. The Adrenal Stress Index, Diagnos-Techs, Kent, WA, 1991:2–5.

7. Podell, RN. Doctor, Why Am I So Tired? (New York: Pharos Books, 1987):151.

8. Ilyia, E. Personal communication. Diagnos-Techs, Kent, WA, 1994.

Chapter 9: The Fitness Factor

1. Clark, SR, et al. Fitness characteristics and perceived exertion in women with fibromyalgia. J Musculoskel Pain 1993; 1 (3/4):191–98.

2. Anonymous. Fitness revolution passing Americans by. The back page 1994; 9 (2):24.

3. Aw, TY, Jones, DP. Nutrient supply and mitochondrial function. Annu Rev Nutr 1989; 9:229–51.

Chapter 10: The Athlete with Fatigue

1. Neiman, DC, Nehlsen-Cannarella, SL, et al. The effects of moderate training on natural killer-cells and acute upper respiratory tract infections. Int J Sports Med 1990; 11 (6):467–73.

2. Watson, RR, et al. Modifications of cellular immune functions in humans by endurance exercise training during beta adrenergic blockade with antenolol or propanolol. Med Sci Sports Ex 1986; 18:95.

3. Surikina, ID. Stress and immunity among athletes. Soviet Sports Rev 1982; 17:198–202.

4. Asgiersson, G, Bellanti, JA. Exercise immunity and infection. Sem

Adolescent Med 987; 3:199–204.

5. Salo, DC. Does swimming make you sick? Swimming World 1989 (October):59.

6. Heath, GW, et al. Exercise and the incidence of upper respiratory tract infections. Med Sci Sports Ex 1991; 23:152–157.

7. Peters, EM, Bateman, ED. Ultramarathon running and upper respiratory tract infections: an epidemiologic survey. SA Med J 1983; 64:582–84.

8. Colgan, M. Sport & Immunity (San Diego, California: The Colgan Institute 1992):1–15.

9. Ibid.

10. Peters, et al. Vitamin C supplementation reduces the incidence of post-race symptoms of upper respiratory tract infection in ultramarathoners. Am J Clin Nutr 1993:57.

11. Sumida, S, Tanaka, K, Kitao, H, Nakadomo, F. Exercise-induced lipid peroxidation and leakage of enzymes before and after vitamin E supplementation. Intl J Biochem 1989; 21:835.

12. Levine, L, et al. Fructose and glucose ingestion and muscle glycogen use during submaximal exercise. J Appl Physiol 1983; 55:1767–71.

13. Moffat, RJ. J Am Diet Assoc 1984; 84:136.

14. Deuster, P, et al. Nutritional intakes and status of highly trained amenorrheic and enmenorrheic women runners. Fertil Steril 1986; 46:636.

15. Budgett, R. The post-viral fatigue syndrome in athletes. In Post-Viral Fatigue Syndrome, Jenkins, R, Mowbray, JF (Eds.) (New York: John Wiley & Sons, 1991):345–362.

16. Budgett, R, et al. The overtraining syndrome/staleness. In Proceedings of the First International Olympic Committee World Congress on Sports Sciences (Colorado Springs, Colorado: U.S. Olympic Committee 1989):118–119.

17. Fitzgerald, L. Exercise and the immune system. Immunol Tod 198; 9:337–39.

18. Dressendorfer, RH. Increased morning heart rate in runners: A valid sign of overtraining? Phys Sports Med 1985; 13 (8):77–86.

19. Ryan, A. Overtraining in athletes: A roundtable. Physician Sports Med 1983; 11:93–100.

20. Aggozzoti, G. Plasma chloroform concentrations in swimmers using indoor swimming pools. Arch Env Hlth 1990; 45 (3):175–179.

21. Nicholson, JP, Case, DB. Carboxyhemoglobin levels in New York City runners. Phys Sports Med 1983; 11:135–138.

22. Clement, DB, Asmundson, RC. Nutritional intake and hematological parameters in endurance runners. Phys Sportsmed 1982; 10 (3):37–43.

23. Selby, GE. When does the athlete need iron? Phys Sports Med 1991; 19 (4):96–102.

24. Shimomuray, et al. Protective effects of coenzyme Q_{10} on exercise-induced muscular injury. Biochem Biophys Res Comm 1991; 176:349–55.

25. Kaminski, M, Boal, R. An effect of ascorbic acid on delayed onset muscle soreness. Pain 1992 (September).

26. Colgan, M. Optimum Sports Nutrition (New York: Advanced Research Press, 1993):247–61.

27. Couzy, F, et al. Zinc metabolism in the athlete: Influence of training, nutrition, and other factors. Int J Sorts Med 1990; 263–266.

28. Sumida, S, Tanaka, K, Kitao, H, Nakadomo, F. Exercise-induced lipid peroxidation and leakage of enzymes before and after vitamin E supplementation. Intl J Biochem 1989; 21:835.

29. Budgett, R. Post-Viral Fatigue Syndrome. Jenkins, R, Mowbray, JF (Eds.) (New York: John Wiley & Sons, 1991):346.

30. Pyke, S, Lew, H, Quintnilha, A. Severe depletion in liver glutathione during physical exercise. Biochem Biophys Res Comm 1986; 139:926–931.

Chapter 11: Posture and Body Mechanics

1. Ebbeling, C.J., Hamill, J., Crussemeyer, J.A. Lower extremity mechanics and energy cost of walking in high-heeled shoes. *J. Orthoped. Sports Phys. Ther.* 1994; 19(4): 190–196.

2. (Donkin, S.W., *Sitting on the Job.* (Boston: Houghton Mifflin Company 1986) 67.

3. Sweere, J (Ed.) Chiropractic Family Practice (Gaithersburg, Maryland: Aspen Publishers, Inc., 1992).

4. Farinelli, E. Effective treatment for chronic fatigue syndrome: Case studies of 70 patients. Monograph, Fort Collins, Colorado 1993.

5. Fidelibus, JC. An overview of neuroimmunomodulation and a possible correlation with musculoskeletal system function. J Man Physiol Ther 1989; 12:289–292.

6. Brennan, PC, Hondras, MA. Priming of neutrophils for enhanced respiratory burst by manipulation of the thoracic spine. Proceedings of the International Conference on Spinal Manipulation 1989; 160–3.

7. Tucker, ME. Osteopathic hands-on approach gains more FP support. Fam Pract News 1994; 25 (6):1.

Chapter 12: Chronic Muscle Pain

1. Goldenberg, DL. Fibromyalgia syndrome: an emerging but controversial condition. JAMA 1987; 257:2782–87.

2. Goldstein, JA. Chronic Fatigue Syndromes: The Limbic Hypothesis (Binghampton, NY: Haworth Press, 1993):71–73.

3. Langer, S. Solved: The Riddle of Illness (New Canaan, Connecticut: Keats Publishing, 1984):143.

4. Smythe, H. Nonarticular rheumatism and psychogenic musculoskeletal syndromes. In McCarty, D (Ed.): Arthritis and Allied Conditions, 10th edition (Philadelphia, Lea & Febiger, 1985):1083–1098.

5. Goldstein, JA. Chronic Fatigue Syndromes: The Limbic Hypothesis (Binghampton, NY: Haworth Press, 1993):71–73.

6. Galland, L. Giardia lamblia infection as a cause of chronic fatigue. J Nutr Med 1990; 1:27–31.

7. Steere, AC, Taylor, E, McHugh, GL, Logigian, EL. The overdiagnosis of Lyme disease. JAMA 1993; 269 (14):1812–16.

8. Lightfoot, RW, et al. Empiric parenteral antibiotic treatment of patients with fibromyalgia and fatigue and positive serologic result for Lyme disease. Ann Intern Med 1993; 119:503–509.

9. Fibromyalgia Network, 23rd edition, Bakersfield, California, 1993.

10. National Research Council. Environmental Neurotoxicology (Washington, D.C.: National Academy Press, 1992):11.

11. Fibromyalgia Network, 23rd edition, Bakersfield, California, 1993.

12. Klein, R, Bansch, M, Berg, PA. Clinical relevance of antibodies against serotonin and gangliosides in patients with primary fibromyalgia syndrome. Psychoneuroendocrinol 1992; 17 (6):593–98.

13. Domingo, JL, Gomez, JM, Llobet, JM, Corbella, J. Comparative effects of several chelating agents on the toxicity, distribution and excretion of aluminum. Hum Toxicol 1988; 7:259–62.

14. Domingo, JL, Gomez, JM, Llobet, JM. Citric, malic and succinic acids as possible alternatives to desferoxamine in aluminum toxicity. J Clin Toxicol 1988; 26:67–79.

15. Davidson, P. Chronic Muscle Pain Syndrome (New York: Villard Books, 1989):142.

16. Hostmark, AT, Lystad, E, Vellar, OD, Hovi, K, Berg, JE. Reduced plasma fibrinogen, serum peroxides, lipids, and apolipoproteins after a 3-week vegetarian diet. Plant Foods Human Nutr 1993; 43:55–61.

17. Moreshead, J, Jaffe, R. Fibromyalgia: clinical success through enhanced host defenses. American Academy of Physical Medicine & Rehabilitation Meeting, Miami, Florida, 1 Nov. 1993.

18. Lee, M. How does IP apply to AIDS patients and those suffering from chronic fatigue? Smokies Digest 1993 (June–August):7.

19. Behan, PO, et al. Effect of high doses of essential fatty acids on the postviral fatigue syndrome. ACTA Neurol Scand 1990; 82:209–16.

20. Bennett, RM. Confounding features of the fibromyalgia syndrome: a current perspective of differential diagnosis. J Rheumatol 1989; 16 (Suppl 19):58–61.

21. Abraham, G, Flechas, J. Management of fibromyalgia: Rationale for the use of magnesium and malic acid. J Nutr Med 992; 3:49–59.

22. Eisinger, J, Zakarian, H, Plantamura, A, Clairet, D, Ayavou, T. Studies of transketolase in chronic pain. J Adv Med 1992; 5 (2):105–113.

23. Eisinger, J, Plantamura, A, Ayavou, T. Glycolysis abnormalities in fibromyalgia. J Am Col Nutr 1994; 13 (2):144–48.

24. Nies, K. Treatment of the fibromyalgia syndrome. J Musculoskel Med 1992; 9 (5):20–26.

25. Yunus, M, Masi, AT, Calabro, JJ, et al. Primary fibromyalgia (fibrositis): Clinical study of 50 patients with matched normal controls. Semin Arthritis Rheum 1981; 11:151–172.

26. Yunus, MB, Masi, AT, Aldag, JC. Ibuprofen in primary fibromyalgia (PFS): A double-blind placebo-controlled study. Arthritis Rheum 1989; 32 (Suppl. 1):R28.

27. Goldenberg, DL, Felson, DT, Dinerman, H. A randomized, controlled trial of amitriptyline and naproxen in the treatment of patients with fibromyalgia. Arthritis Rheum 1986; 29:1371–1377.

28. Caruso, I, Puttinin, PS, Cazzola, M, Azzolini, V. Double-blind study of 5-hydroxy tryptophan versus placebo in the treatment of primary fibromyalgia syndrome. J Inter Med Res 1990; 18:201–209.

29. Deluze, C, et al. Electroacupuncture in fibromyalgia: results of a controlled trial. Br Med J 1992; 305:1249–52.

30. Fischer, P, Greenwood, A, Huskission, EC, Turner, P, Belon, P. Effect of homeopathic treatment on fibrositis (primary fibromyalgia). Br Med J 1989; 299:365–66.

31. McKain, GA. Role of physical fitness training in the fibrositis/fibromyalgia syndrome. Am J Med 1986; 81:73–77.

Chapter 13: Infections That May Cause Fatigue

1. McKeown, T. The Role of Medicine: Dream, Mirage or Nemesis (Princeton, NJ: Princeton University Press, 1979):107.

2. Stewart, A. Nutrition and the post-viral fatigue syndrome, In Jenkins, R, Mowbray, J (Eds.), Post-Viral Fatigue Syndrome (New York: John Wiley & Sons, 1991):385–92.

3. Behan, PO, Behan, WMH, Horrobin, DF. Placebo-controlled trial of n-3 and n-6 essential fatty acids in the treatment of post-viral fatigue syndrome. Acta Neurologica Scand 1990; 82:209–16.

4. Crook, WG. Chronic Fatigue Syndrome and the Yeast Connection (Jackson, Tennessee: Professional Books, 1993).

5. Ibid, 340.

6. Ibid, 319.

7. Steere, AC, Taylor, E, McHugh, GL, Logigian, EL. The overdiagnosis of Lyme disease. JAMA 1993; 269 (14):1812–16.

8. Brenner, C, O'Donnell, JS, Gabriel, MC. Scientist challenges Steere's methods and conclusions. The Lyme Times 1993; 11:43–46.

9. Nocton, J, et al. Detection of Borrelia burgdorferi DNA by polymerase chain reaction in synovial fluid from patients with Lyme arthritis. N Engl J Med 1994; 330:229–34.

10. Galland, L. Giardia lamblia infection as a cause of chronic fatigue. J Nutr Med 1990; 1:27–31.

11. Galland, L, Lee, M. High frequency giardiasis in patients with chronic digestive complaints. (Abstract) Am J Gastroenterol 1989; 84:1181.

12. Lee, MJ, Barrie, SA. Evaluation of random, purged, and swab specimens for the detection of fecal parasites. Presented at the American Society of Microbiology 93rd General Meeting, Atlanta, Georgia, May 16–20, 1993.

13. Galland, L. The effect of intestinal microbes on systemic immunity. In Jenkins, R, Mowbray, J (Eds.), Post-Viral Fatigue Syndrome (New York: John Wiley & Sons, 1991).

Chapter 14: Antibiotic Overuse

1. Crook, WG. Chronic Fatigue Syndrome and the Yeast Connection (Jackson, Tennessee: Professional Books, 1993):319.

2. Ali, M. Clinician of the Month. Preventive Medicine Update, December 1993.

3. Bauman, DS, Hagglund, HE. Polysystem chronic complainers. J Adv Med 1991; 4 (1).

4. Cohen, ML. Epidemiology of drug resistance: implications for a post-antimicrobial era. Science 1992; 257:1050–1055.

5. Neu, HC. The crisis in antibiotic resistance. Science 1992; 257:1064–1073.

6. Fisher, JA. The Plague Makers (New York: Simon & Schuster, 1994):53–76.

7. Hunnisett, A, Howard, J, Davies, S. Gut fermentation (or the "auto-brewery") syndrome: a new clinical test with initial observations and discussion of clinical and biochemical implications. J Nutr Med 1990; 1:33–38.

8. Galland, L. Dysbiosis Patterns, In Application Guide (Asheville, North Carolina: Great Smokies Diagnostic Laboratory, 1992).

9. Comprehensive Digestive Stool Analysis. Great Smokies Diagnostic Laboratory, Application Guide, 1993.

10. Schmidt, MA, Smith, LS, Sehnert, KW. Beyond Antibiotics (Berkeley, California: North Atlantic Books, 1994).

Chapter 16: Prescription Drugs That Make You Tired

1. Podell, R. Doctor, Why Am I So Tired? (New York: Pharos Books, 1987):217–223.

2. Stoff, JA, Pellegrino, CR. Chronic Fatigue Syndrome: The Hidden Epidemic. Revised Edition (New York: Harper Perennial, 1992).

3. Roe, DA, Campbell, TC, eds. Drugs and Nutrients: The Interactive Effects. New York: Marcel Dekker, Inc.; 1984.

4. Roe, DA. Handbook: Interactions of Selected Drugs and Nutrients in Patients (Chicago, Illinois: The American Dietetic Association, 1982).

5. Roe, DA. Drug-Induced Nutritional Deficiencies (Westport, Connecticut: Avi Publishing, 1985).

6. Roe, DA. Diet and Drug Interactions (New York, NY: Van Nostrand Reinhold, 1989).

7. Stephenson, J. Detox is crucial in chronic daily headache. Fam Pract News 1993, July 1.

8. Physician's Desk Reference (Oradell, New Jersey: Medical Economics Company, 1993).

9. Podell, R. Doctor, Why Am I So Tired? (New York: Pharos Books, 1987):217–223.

Chapter 17: Tired or Toxic

1. Carter-Pokras, O, Brody, D, Murphy, RS. Selected pesticide residues and metabolites in urine from a survey of the U.S. general population. J Tox Env Hlth 1992; 37:277–291.

2. Feldman, R. Am J Indust Med, 1980.

3. Agency for Toxic Substances and Disease Registry. Methylene chloride toxicity. Am Fam Phys 1993; 4:1159–1165.

4. Buist, RA. Chronic fatigue syndrome and chemical overload. Intl Clin Nutr Rev 1988; 8 (4):173–175.

5. Buscher, DS. Chronic fatigue syndrome relation to chemical sensitivities. Well Mind Association Meeting, Seattle, Washington, December 1992.

6. National Research Council. Environmental Neurotoxicology (Washington, D.C.: National Academy Press, 1992):11.

7. Wallace, L, Pellizzari, E, et al. Exposure to volatile organic compounds: Direct measurement in breathing-zone air, drinking water, food, and exhaled breath. Env Res 1984; 35:193–211.

8. Gammage, RB, White, DA, Bupta, KC. Residential measurements of high volatility organics and their sources. Indoor Air, Swedish Council for Building Research, Stockholm, Sweden, 1984; 4:157–162.

9. Gammage, RB, Kaye, SV. Indoor Air and Human Health (Boca Raton, Florida: Lewis Publishers, 1984):331–411.

10. Rogers, S. Tired or Toxic (Syracuse, New York: Prestige Publishers, 1990):75.

11. McConnachie, PR, Zahalsky, AC. Immune alterations in humans exposed to the termiticide technical chlordane. Arch Env Hlth 1992; 47 (4):295–301.

12. Rogers, S. Tired or Toxic (Syracuse, New York: Prestige Publishers, 1990):75.

13. van Raaji, JAGM, et al, Neurotoxic chlorinated hydrocarbons penetrate the blood-brain barrier possibly by binding to thyroid hormone transport proteins. Neurotoxicology 1991; 12 (4):818.

14. Edling, C, et al. Occupational exposure to organic solvents as a cause of sleep apnea. Br J Indust Med 1993; 50:276–279.

15. Lindelof, B., Almkvist, O., Crothe, C.J. Sleep disturbances and exposure to organic solvents. Arch Env Hlth 1992; 47(2): 104–106.

16. National Research Council. Environmental Neurotoxicology (Wash-

ington, D.C.: National Academy Press, 1992):11.

17. Dudley, D. Personal communication. Seattle, Washington, 1994.

18. Schwartz, G. Personal communication. Tucson, Arizona, 1993.

19. Jaffe, RM. Personal communication. Reston, Virginia, 1994.

20. Ali, M. Clinician of the Month. Preventive Medicine Update, December 1993.

21. Danersund, A, Lindvall, A, Lindh, U. Elemental profiles in 25 patients with chronic disease. In Trace Elements in Human Health. Presentation Abstracts. Amsterdam, Holland, August 1993.

22. Stejskal, V. Immunological reactions to metals in patients with chronic fatigue syndrome. International Symposium on Functional Medicine. Presentation Abstracts. Palm Springs, California, April 1994.

23. Rogers, S. Tired or Toxic (Syracuse, New York: Prestige Publishers, 1990):143.

Chapter 18: Airborne Allergy

1. Rogers, S. The EI Syndrome (Syracuse, NY: Prestige Publishers, 1986):142–147.

2. Mendell, MJ, Smith, AH. Consistent pattern of elevated symptoms in air-conditioned office buildings: a reanalysis of epidemiologic studies. Am J Pub Hlth 1990; 80:1193–1199.

Chapter 19: Light

1. Chernoff, R. Geriatric Nutrition (Gaithersburg, Maryland: Aspen Publishers, 1991):29.

2. Liberman, J. Light: Medicine of the Future (Santa Fe, New Mexico: Bear & Company, 1991):54–5.

3. Szent-Gyorgyi, A. Bioelectronics (New York: Academic Press, 1968).

4. Cross, M. New techniques help cure winter blues. The Valley Vantage, 1990 (Feb. 1):5.

5. Rosenthal, N. Seasonal affective disorder. Brain/Mind Bulletin 1986; 11 (13):3.

6. Raitiere, MN. Clinical evidence for thyroid dysfunction in patients with seasonal affective disorder. Psychoneuroendocrinol 1992; 17 (2/3):231–41.

7. Hill, MA. Light, circadian rhythms, and mood disorders: a review. Ann Clin Psychiatry 1992; 4:131–146.

8. Hill, MA. Winter depression. Your Health 1993; 14 (1):1–2.

Chapter 20: Sleep and Rest

1. Anonymous. Natural Health 1993 (July/Aug):21.

2. Podell, R. Doctor, Why Am I So Tired? (New York: Pharos Books, 1987):217–223.

3. Hale, E. Suits argue fatigue puts public at risk. USA Today (October 1, 1993).

4. Edling, C, et al. Occupational exposure to organic solvents as a cause of sleep apnea. Br J Indust Med 1993; 50:276–79.

5. Davis, W, Ziady, F. Magnesium and Sleep. Presented at the Second International Symposium on Magnesium, Montreal, 1976.

6. Braverman, ER, Pfeiffer, CC. The Healing Nutrients Within (New Canaan, Connecticut: Keats Publishing, 1987).

7. Lindelof, B., Almkvist, O., Crothe, C.J. Sleep disturbances and exposure to organic solvents. Arch Env Hlth 1992; 47(2): 104–106.

8. National Research Council. Environmental Neurotoxicology (Washington, D.C.: National Academy Press, 1992):11.

9. Davis, W, Ziady, F. Magnesium and Sleep. Presented at the Second International Symposium on Magnesium, Montreal, 1976.

10. Lindahl, O, Lindwall, L. Double blind study of a valerian preparation. Pharmacol Biochem Behav 1989; 32 (4):1065–66.

11. Tisserand, R. The Art of Aromatherapy (Rochester, Vermont: Healing Arts Press, 1977):301.

12. Schnaubelt, K. Personal communication, 1993.

Chapter 21: Circumstantial Fatigue

1. Women abused as kids found in poorer health. The New York Times (August, 1990).

2. Podell, R. Doctor, Why Am I So Tired? (New York: Pharos Books, 1987):108–115.

Chapter 22: Psychological Factors

1. Werbach, M. Nutritional Influences on Mental Illness (Tarzana, California: Third Line Press, 1991):123–151.

2. Slagle, P. The Way Up from Down (New York: Random House, 1987):68.

3. Jaffe, RM, Kruesi, OR. The biochemical-immunology window: A molecular view of psychiatric case management. J Appl Nutr 1992; 44 (2):26–42.

4.Slagle, P. The Way Up from Down (New York: Random House, 1987):68.

5. Jaffe, RM, Kruesi, OR. The biochemical-immunology window: A molecular view of psychiatric case management. J Appl Nutr 1992; 44 (2):26–42.

6. Nasr, S, et al. Concordance of atopic and affective disorders. J Affective Disord 1981; 3:291.

7. King, DS. Can allergic exposure provoke psychological symptoms? A double-blind test. Biol Psych 1981; 16 (1):3–19.

8. Haggerty, JJ, et al. Subclinical hypothyroidism: A modifiable risk factor for depression. Am J Psych 1993; 150:508–510.

9. Tintera, J. Hypoadrenia. N Y State J Med 1955; 55 (13).

10. Hoffer, A. Allergy, depression and tricyclic antidepressants. J Orthomol Psychol 1980; 9 (3):164–70.

11. Podell, R. Doctor, Why Am I So Tired? (New York: Pharos Books, 1987):217–223.

12. Osborn, G. Personal communication on Prozac and chronic fatigue, 1994.

13. Podell, R. Doctor, Why Am I So Tired? (New York: Pharos Books, 1987):217–223.

14. Boyce, TW, et al. Influence of life events and family routines on childhood respiratory tract illness. Pediatrics 1977; 60 (4):609–615.

15. Meyer, RJ, Haggerty, RJ. Streptococcal infections in families. Pediatrics 1962; 4:539–49.

16. Cohen, S, Tyrrell, D, Smith, A. Psychological stress and susceptibility to the common cold. New Engl J Med 1991; 325:606–12.

17. Henrotte, JG, et al. Blood and urinary magnesium, zinc, calcium, free fatty acids, and catecholamines in Type A and Type B subjects. Journal of the American College of Nutrition 1985; 4:165–172.

18. Crook, WG. Chronic Fatigue Syndrome and the Yeast Connection (Jackson, Tennessee: Professional Books, 1993):253.

19. Adler, G. The physician and the hypochondrial patient. New Engl J Med 1981 (June 4):1394–96.

20. Chopra, D. Ageless Body, Timeless Mind (New York: Harmony Books, 1993).

21. Justice, B. Who Gets Sick: How Thoughts, Moods and Beliefs Can Affect Your Health (Los Angeles: J.P. Tarcher, 1988).

22. Peterson, C. Explanatory style as a risk factor for illness. Cognitive

Therapy Research 1988; 12:117–30. See also Peterson, C. Journal of Personality and Social Psychology.

23. Sobel, D, Ornstein, R. Healthy Pleasures (Reading, Massachusetts: Addison Wesley, 1989):168.

24. Seligman, MEP. Learned Optimism (New York: Alfred A. Knopf, 1991):167–184.

25. Ibid, 174.

Chapter 23: Motherhood and Fatigue

1. Pop, VJM, et al. Microsomal antibodies during gestation in relation to postpartum thyroid dysfunction and depression. ACTA Endocrinol 1993; 129:26–30.

Chapter 24: Boosting Energy and Restoring Balance

1. Newberne, PM, Williams, G. Nutritional influences on the course of infections. In Dunlop, RH, Moon, HW. Resistance to Infectious Disease (Saskatoon, Canada: Saskatoon Modern Press, 1970):93.

2. Neiman, DC, Nehlsen-Cannarella, SL, Markoff, PA, et al. The effects of moderate exercise training on natural killer-cells and acute upper respiratory tract infections. Int J Sports Med 1990; 11 (6):467–73.

3. Peters, EM, Bateman, ED. Ultramarathon running and upper respiratory tract infections: An epidemiology survey. SA Med J 1983; 64:582–584.

4. Moskowitz, H. Hiding in the Hammond report. Hospital Practice 1975; 8:35–39.

5. Batmanghelhidj, F. Your Body's Many Cries for Water. Falls Church, Virginia: Global Health Solutions, Inc., 1992.

Chapter 25: Detoxification

1. Rigden, S, Bralley, JA, Bland, JS. Management of chronic fatigue symptoms by tailored nutritional intervention using a program designed to support hepatic detoxification. Unpublished report, 1993.

2. Casarett and Doull's Toxicology: The Basic Science of Poisons. Amdur, MO, Doull, J, Klassen, CD (Eds.) (New York: Pergamon Press, 1991):16–17.

3. Rigden, S, Bralley, JA, Bland, JS. Management of chronic fatigue symptoms by tailored nutritional intervention using a program designed to support hepatic detoxification. Unpublished report, 1993.

4. Ibid.

Chapter 26: Breath and Energy

1. Chia, M, Chia, M. Transforming Stress Into Vitality (Huntington, New York: Healing Tao Books, 1985).

2. Chia, M, Chia, M. Chi Nei Tsang: Internal Organs Chi Massage (Huntington, New York: Healing Tao Books, 1986).

3. Collinge, W. Recovering from Chronic Fatigue Syndrome (New York: Body Press/Perigree, 1993).

Chapter 27: The Case of Dr. Tom

1. Bralley, JA. Amino acids and chronic fatigue. Personal communication, 1993.

2. Douglas, SD. Cells involved in immune responses. In Fudenberg, HH, Stites, DP, Caldwell, JL, Wells, JV. (Eds.) Basic & Clinical Immunology, 3rd edition (Los Altos, California: Lange Medical Publications, 1980)96–114.

3. Bucci, LR. A functional analytical technique for monitoring nutrient status and repletion. Am Clin Lab 1993; 12 (6):8.

4. Window on SpectraCell. SpectraCell Laboratories 1994 (Spring):3–4.

5. Rogers, S. Tired or Toxic? (Syracuse, NY: Prestige Publishers, 1989):143.

Additional information on laboratory testing.

Werbach, M. Nutritional Influences on Illness (Tarzana, California: Third Line Press, 1988):467–477.

Chapter 28: Questions You Might Ask

1. Anonymous. Women abused as kids found in poorer health. The New York Times (August 1990).

2. Jaffe, RM. Chronic fatigue protocol: clinical suggestions. Intl Clin Nutr Rev 1991; 11:85–91.

3. Jaffe, RM. Personal communication, 1993.

Index

About the Author

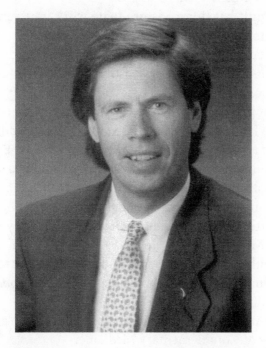

MICHAEL A. SCHMIDT is a clinician, scientist, and medical educator whose work ranges broadly from the nutritional biochemistry of the brain and immune system to psychobiology and mind-body medicine. Over the past 15 years, he has helped to advance the field of functional medicine.

While studying medicine at Russian State Medical University he had the opportunity to work with Dr. Yevgeny Gusev, Chairman of the Department of Neurology and Neurosurgery and with Dr. Alexander Archakov, Chairman of the Department of Biochemistry, both of the Russian Academy of Medical Sciences. He transferred from the medical school to pursue a Ph.D. in psychoneurobiology and nutritional biochemistry. As part of his doctoral work he has studied in collaboration with physicians and scientists at NASA (National Aeronautics and Space Administration) and elsewhere. Part of his work has involved looking at nutrient modulators of brain and immune function and also the way in which psychological factors influence nutrient chemistry.

Dr. Schmidt has done postgraduate work in psychoneuroimmunology under faculty of the Center for Mind-Body Medicine at Harvard Medical School and has also studied medical imagery through the American Imagery Institute at the University of Wisconsin School of Medicine.

He is a nutritional biochemist and licensed clinical nutritionist, who teaches laboratory diagnostics at the graduate and postgraduate level. He is a former Visiting Professor of Applied Biochemistry and Clinical Nutrition, at Northwestern College, and has lectured in nutritional neuroscience and immunology. Dr. Schmidt is on the Scientific Council of the International and American Association of Clinical Nutritionists. While an associate of Dr. Jeffrey Bland at the Functional Medicine Research Center in Gig Harbor, Washington he helped author clinical textbooks and teaching materials for physicians including the recent *Clinical Nutrition: A Functional Approach.* He is a contributing author to *The Textbook of Complementary Medicine,* which was edited by the National Institutes of Health Director of the Office of Complementary Medicine.

Dr. Schmidt has written numerous books on integrated medicine for the general reader including *Beyond Antibiotics* and *Smart Fats.* He has appeared on many national radio and television shows and was recently a featured guest on a PBS Special about nutrition in depression and anxiety. He was born in Minnesota and makes his home in Washington state.